Vegetarian Recipes for Every Occasion

Learn How to Cook the Vegetarian Way and Surprise Your Guests with Super-Tasty and Healthy Recipes

America Best Recipes

Table of Contents

Breakfast 5

    Kale and Spinach Smoothie 5

    Peanut Butter and Coffee Smoothie 6

    Broccoli and Quinoa Breakfast Patties 7

    Sweet Potato Breakfast Hash 9

    Scrambled Eggs with Aquafaba 11

    Enchilada Breakfast Casserole...............................13

    Sweet Crepes 15

    Tomato and Asparagus Quiche...............................16

    Ultimate Breakfast Sandwich 18

    Breakfast Barley 20

    Almond Honey Quinoa 22

Lunch 24

    Fresh Bell Pepper Basil Pizza..................................24

    Keto Cheesy Broccoli & Cauliflower Rice 28

    Low-Carb Vegetarian Greek Briam...........................30

    Cauliflower Confetti Kale Pecan Salad 33

    Roasted Mushroom and Walnut Cauliflower Grits...................35

    Mexican cauliflower patties....................................38

    Mediterranean "Pasta" 41

    Grilled Halloumi Bruschetta 43

    Zucchini Ricotta Tart...45

Soups and Salads..48

    Cucumber, Mango, and Barley Salad 48

    Greek Green Bean Salad with Feta and Tomatoes...................50

    Quick Edamame Salad 52

    Green Bean and Potato Salad 54

    Lemon Millet Vegetable Salad 56

Crisp Green Bean Salad 58

Broccoli and Noodle Salad 61

Greek Lentil Salad 63

Red Quinoa and Avocado Salad 66

Dinner 68

Baked Crimini Mushrooms and Red Potatoes......... 68

Baked Button Mushroom and Summer Squash 71

Rutabagas Curry 74

Baked Brussel Sprouts & Red Onion Glazed with Balsamic
Vinegar 77

Roasted Savoy Cabbage and Vidalia Onion 80

Baked Watercress and Summer Squash 82

Curried Kale and Rutabaga 84

Buttered Potatoes and Spinach 85

Roasted Vegan-Buttered Mustard Greens Carrots 88

Smoky Roasted Swiss Chard and Cauliflower 89

Sweets 91

Chocolate Chip Mini Muffins 91

Pumpkin Spice Coffee Muffins 93

Blueberry Cream Muffins 95

Apple Pumpkin Muffins 97

Pineapple Zucchini Muffins 100

Blackberries Compote 102

Raspberry-Vanilla Barley Pudding 103

Nectarines Cobbler 105

Hazelnuts Corn Syrup Mousse 107

Coconut Brownies 109

Breakfast

Kale and Spinach Smoothie

Preparation time: 5 minutes Cooking time: 0 minute

Servings: 1

Ingredients:

1 cup spinach

1 cup kale

1 frozen banana 3 small dates, pitted

1 1/4 cup almond milk, unsweetened

1 scoop of vanilla protein powder

1 teaspoon cinnamon

Directions:

Place all the ingredients in the order in a food processor or blender and then pulse for 2 to 3 minutes at high speed until smooth. Pour the smoothie into a glass and then serve.

Peanut Butter and Coffee Smoothie

Preparation time: 5 minutes Cooking time: 0 minute

Servings: 1

Ingredients:

2 small frozen banana

1/2 teaspoon ground turmeric

1 tablespoon chia seeds

1 scoop of chocolate protein powder

2 tablespoons Peanut Butter

1 cup strong coffee, brewed

Directions:

Place all the ingredients in the order in a food processor or blender and then pulse for 2 to 3 minutes at high speed until smooth. Pour the smoothie into a glass and then serve.

Broccoli and Quinoa Breakfast Patties

Preparation time: 5 minutes Cooking time: 6 minutes
Servings: 4

Ingredients:

1 cup cooked quinoa, cooked

1/2 cup shredded broccoli florets

1/2 cup shredded carrots

2 cloves of garlic, minced

2 teaspoon parsley

1 1/2 teaspoon onion powder

1 1/2 teaspoon garlic powder

1/3 teaspoon salt

1/4 teaspoon black pepper

1/2 cup bread crumbs, gluten-free

2 tablespoon coconut oil 2 flax eggs

Directions:

Prepare patties and for this, place all the ingredients in a large bowl, except for oil and stir until well combined and then shape the mixture into patties. Take a skillet pan, place it over medium heat, add oil and when hot, add prepared patties in it and cook for 3 minutes per side until golden brown and crispy. Serve patties with vegan sour creams.

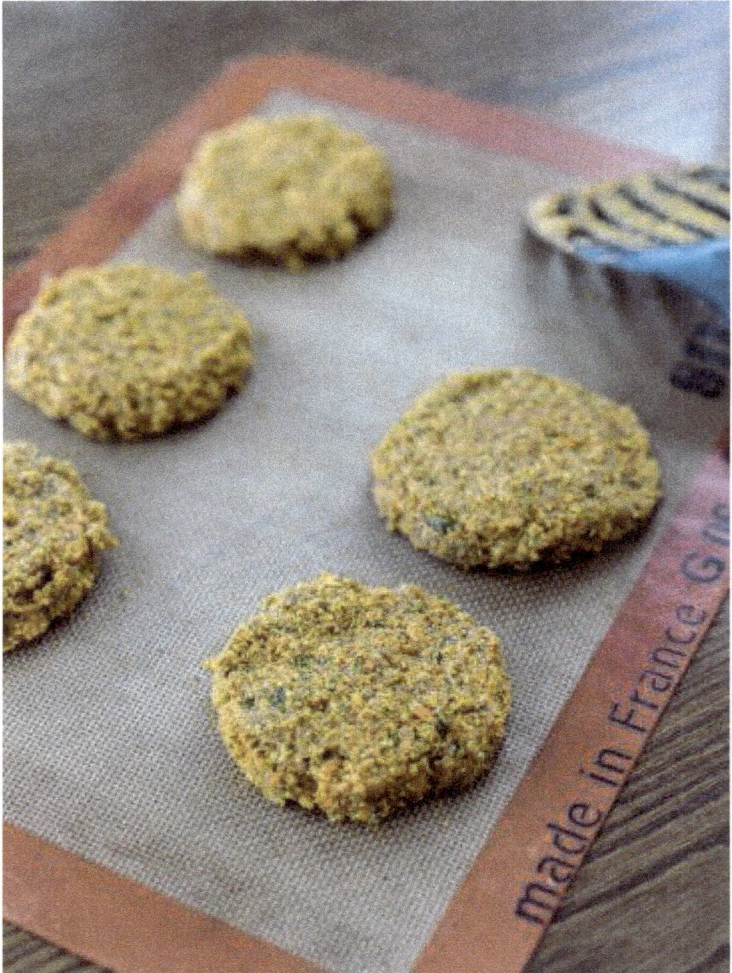

Sweet Potato Breakfast Hash

Preparation time: 5 minutes Cooking time: 28 minutes

Servings: 4

Ingredients:

4 cups cubed sweet potatoes, peeled

1/2 teaspoon sea salt

1/2 teaspoon turmeric

1/2 teaspoon cumin

1 teaspoon smoked paprika

2 cups diced white onion

2 cloves of garlic, peeled, minced

1/4 cup chopped cilantro

1 tablespoon coconut oil

½ cup vegan guacamole, for serving

1 ½ cup pica de Gallo

Directions:

Take a skillet pan, place it over medium heat, add oil. When it melts, add onion, potatoes, and garlic, season with salt, paprika, turmeric, and cumin, stir and cook for 25 minutes until potatoes are slightly caramelized. Then remove the pan from heat, add cilantro and distribute evenly between serving plates. Top the sweet potato hash with guacamole and pico de gallo and then serve.

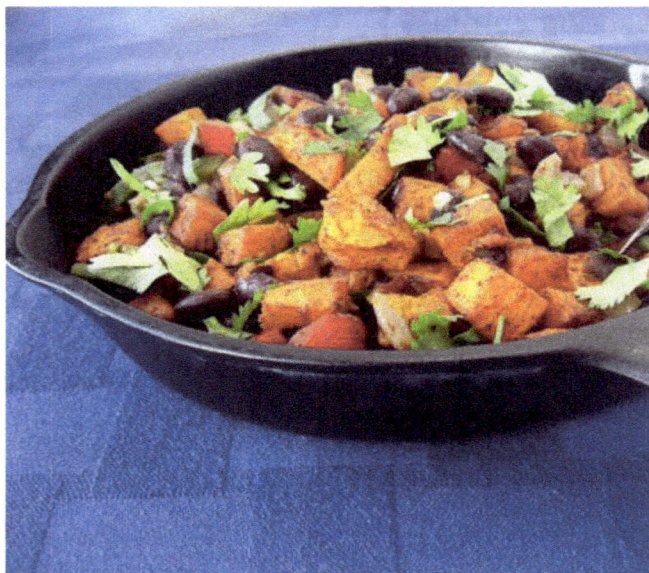

Scrambled Eggs with Aquafaba

Preparation time: 5 minutes Cooking time: 15 minutes

Servings: 2

Ingredients:

6 ounces tofu, firm, pressed, drained

1/2 cup aquafaba

1 1/2 tablespoons olive oil

1 tablespoon nutritional yeast

1/4 teaspoon black salt

1/8 teaspoon ground turmeric

1/4 teaspoon ground black pepper

Directions:

Take a food processor, add tofu, yeast, black pepper, salt, and turmeric, then pour in aquafaba and olive oil and pulse for 1 minute until smooth. Take a skillet pan, place it over medium heat, and when hot, add tofu mixture and cook for 1 minute. Cover the pan, continue cooking for 3 minutes, then uncover the pan and pull the mixture across the pan with a wooden spoon until soft forms. Continue cooking for 10 minutes until resembles soft scrambled eggs, folding tofu mixture gently and heat over medium heat, then remove the pan from heat and season with salt and black pepper to taste. Serve straight away.

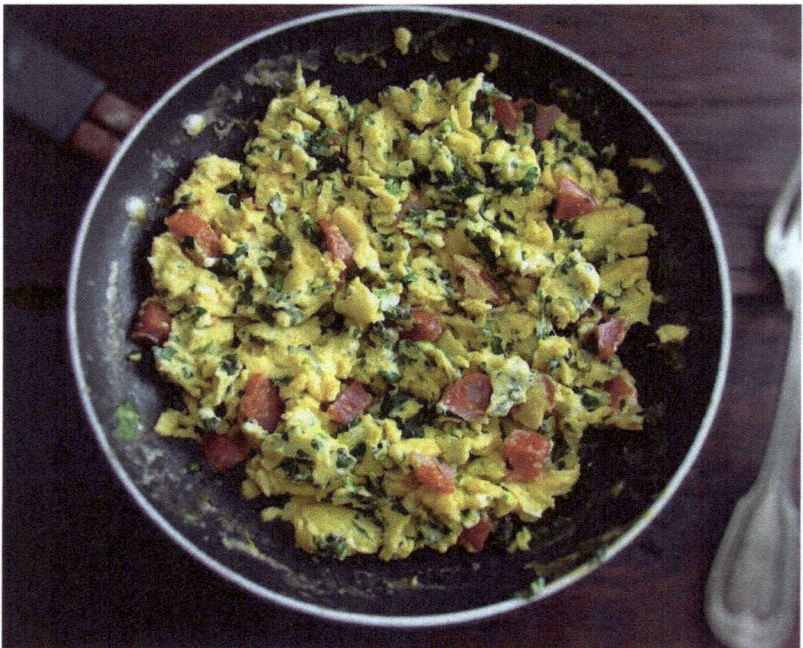

Enchilada Breakfast Casserole

Preparation time: 10 minutes Cooking time: 25 minutes

Servings: 8

Ingredients:

15 ounces cooked corn

1 batch of vegan breakfast eggs

15 ounces cooked pinto beans

3 medium zucchini, sliced into rounds

10 ounces of vegan cheddar cheese, shredded

24 ounces red enchilada sauce

12 corn tortillas, cut into wedges

Shredded lettuce for serving

Vegan sour cream for serving

Directions:

Take a skillet pan, grease it with oil and press the vegan breakfast eggs into the bottom of the pan in an even layer. Spread with 1/3 of enchilada sauce, then sprinkle with half of the cheese and cover with half of the tortilla wedges. Cover the wedges with 1/3 of the sauce, then layer with beans, corn, and zucchini, cover with remaining tortilla wedges, and spread the remaining sauce on top. Cover the pan with lid, place it over medium heat and cook for 25 minutes until cheese had melted, zucchini is tender, and sauce is bubbling. When done, let the casserole stand for 10 minutes, top with lettuce and sour cream, then cut the casserole into wedges, and serve.

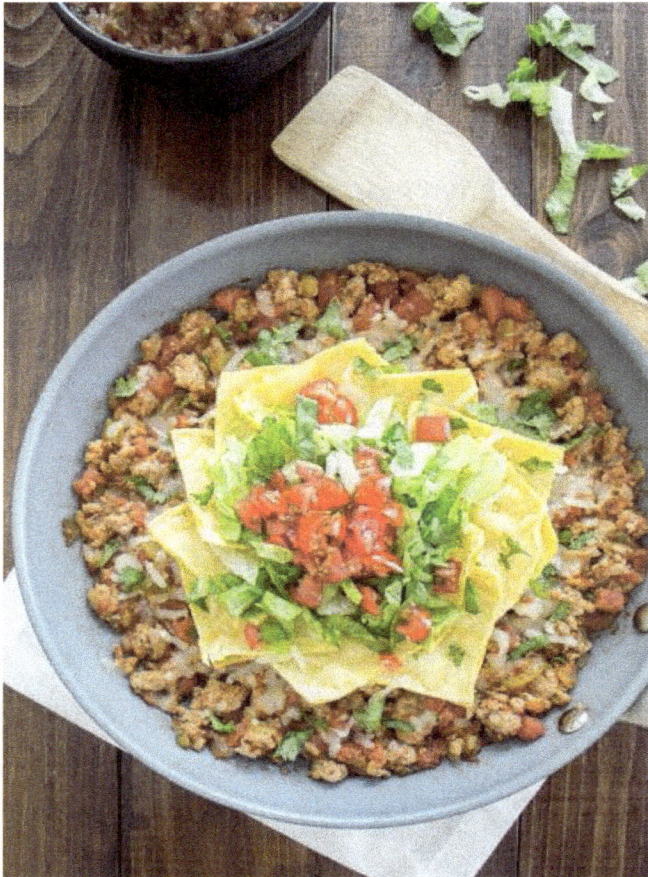

Sweet Crepes

Preparation time: 5 minutes Cooking time: 8 minutes Servings: 5

Ingredients:

1 cup of water

1 banana

1/2 cup oat flour

1/2 cup brown rice flour

1 teaspoon baking powder

1 tablespoon coconut sugar

1/8 teaspoon salt

Directions:

Take a blender, place all the ingredients except for sugar and salt and pulse for 1 minute until smooth. Take a skillet pan, place it over medium- high heat, grease it with oil and when hot, pour in ¼ cup of batter, spread it as thin as possible, and cook for 2 to 3 minutes per side until golden brown. Cook remaining crepes in the same manner, then sprinkle with sugar and salt and serve.

Tomato and Asparagus Quiche

Preparation time: 40 minutes Cooking time: 35 minutes Servings: 12

Ingredients:

For the Dough:

2 cups whole wheat flour

1/2 teaspoon salt

¾ cup vegan margarine

1/3 cup water

For the Filling:

14 oz silken tofu 6 cherry tomatoes, halved 2 green onions, cut into rings 10 sun-dried tomatoes, in oil, chopped 7 oz green asparagus, diced 1 1/2 tablespoons herbs de Provence 1 tablespoon cornstarch 1 teaspoon turmeric 3 tablespoons olive oil

Directions:

Switch on the oven, then set it to 350 degrees F and let it preheat. Pre the dough and take a bowl, place all the ingredients for it, beat until incorporated, knead for 5 minutes until smooth, and refrigerate the dough for 30 minutes. Meanwhile, take a skillet pan, place it over medium heat, add 1 tablespoon oil and when hot, add green onion and cook for 2 minutes, set aside until required.

Place a pot half full wit salty water over medium heat, bring it to boil, add asparagus and boil for 3 minutes until tender, drain and set aside until required. Take a medium bowl, add tofu along with herbs de Provence, starch, turmeric, and oil, whisk until smooth and then fold in tomatoes, green onion, and asparagus until mixed.

Divide the prepared dough into twelve sections, take a muffin tray, line it twelve cups with baking cups, and then press a dough ball at the bottom of each cup and up. Fill the cups with prepared tofu mixture, top with tomatoes, and bake for 35 minutes until cooked. Serve straight away.

Ultimate Breakfast Sandwich

Preparation time: 40 minutes Cooking time: 10 minutes

Servings: 4

Ingredients:

For the Tofu:

12 ounces tofu, extra-firm, pressed, drain

1/2 teaspoon garlic powder

1 teaspoon liquid smoke

2 tablespoons nutritional yeast

1 teaspoon Sriracha sauce

2 tablespoons soy sauce

2 tablespoons olive oil

2 tablespoons water

For the Vegan Breakfast Sandwich:

1 large tomato, sliced

4 English muffins, halved, toasted

1 avocado, mashed

Directions:

Prepare tofu, and for this, cut tofu into four slices and set aside. Stir together remaining ingredients of tofu, pour the mixture into a bag, add tofu pieces, toss until coated and marinate for 30 minutes. Take a skillet pan, place it over medium-high heat, add tofu slices along with the marinade and cook for 5 minutes per side. Prepare sandwich and for this, spread mashed avocado on the inner of the muffin, top with a slice of tofu, layer with a tomato slice and then serve.

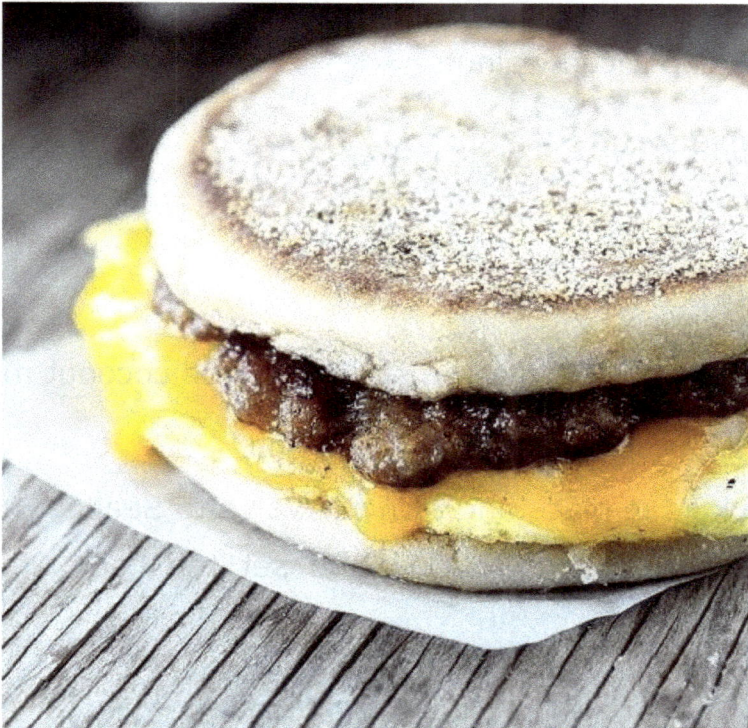

Breakfast Barley

Prep time: 10 min Cooking Time: 15 min Serve: 4

Ingredients

½ cup barley rinsed

1/2 coconut milk

Kosher salt

1/8 teaspoon ground nutmeg

½ cup generous mixed blackberries, raspberries, and blueberries

1/8 cup sliced walnuts

Maple syrup

Instructions

Put the barley in the Instant Pot. Add coconut milk, salt, and the nutmeg.

Lock lid in place and turn the valve to Sealing. Press the Pressure Cooker button and set the cook time for 5 minutes at High Pressure.

Let the steam release naturally for 12 minutes, then turn the valve to Venting to release any residual steam quickly. Carefully remove the lid and fluff the barley with a fork.

To serve, divide the barley evenly among four bowls. Top the barley with the berries and walnuts, drizzle with maple syrup, and serve right away.

Nutrition Facts

Calories 389, Total Fat 19.6g, Saturated Fat 13.1g, Cholesterol 0mg, Sodium 15mg, Total Carbohydrate 49.7g, Dietary Fiber 9.7g, Total Sugars 8.5g, Protein 8.2g

Almond Honey Quinoa

Prep time: 10 min Cooking Time: 05 min Serve: 2

Ingredients

½ cup quinoa

1 1/2 cups water

½ tablespoon coconut oil

1/16 teaspoon salt

½ cup almond butter

1 cup diced banana

1 tablespoon honey

1/8 teaspoon ground cinnamon

Instructions

Combine quinoa, water, coconut oil, salt in an Instant Pot.

Lock lid in place and turn the valve to Sealing. Press the Pressure Cooker button and set the cook time for 5 minutes at High Pressure.

Open the Instant Pot to use natural pressure release.

Stir in almond butter.

Divide quinoa mixture among 2 bowls. Top with banana, and drizzle with honey. Sprinkle with cinnamon, and serve immediately.

Nutrition Facts

Calories 305, Total Fat 8g, Saturated Fat 2.4g, Cholesterol 8mg, Sodium 101mg, Total Carbohydrate 53.9g, Dietary Fiber 5.4g , Total Sugars 18g, Protein 7.7g

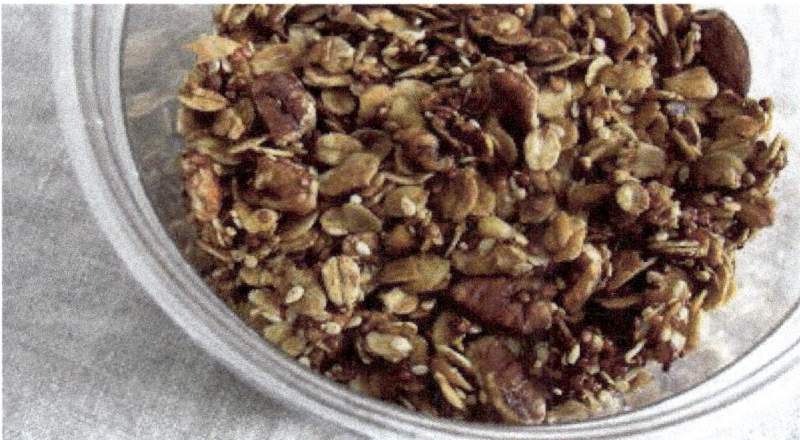

Lunch
Fresh Bell Pepper Basil Pizza

Servings: 2 Fresh Pizza Base

Toppings

6 ounces mozzarella cheese

½ cup almond flour

2 tablespoons psyllium husk 2 tablespoons cream
cheese

2 tablespoons fresh Parmesan cheese 1 large egg

1 teaspoon Italian seasoning

½ teaspoon salt

½ teaspoon pepper

4 ounces shredded cheddar cheese

Instructions

Preheat oven to 400F. Start by measuring out all of your dry spices and flours in a bowl. 1/2 cup Almond Flour, 2 tbsp. Psyllium Husk, 2 tbsp. Fresh Parmesan Cheese, 1 tsp. Italian Seasoning, 1/2 tsp. Salt, and 1/2 tsp. Pepper.

Measure out 6 oz. Mozzarella Cheese into a bowl.

Microwave the cheese for 40-50 seconds until it's completely melted and pliable with your hands. Add 2 tbsp. Cream Cheese to the top.

Add 1 egg to the dry ingredients and mix together a little bit. Add the melted mozzarella cheese and cream cheese to the egg and dry ingredients and mix everything together. Don't mind getting your hands dirty here – they'll be the best tool for the job. You'll get a bit messy, but it'll be oh so worth it in the end. Break the dough into 2 equal (or almost equal) portions. Roll the dough out quite thin – a little under 1/4". Here, you can use the top of a pot or other large round object to cut out your pizza base. You can form the circles by hand, but I'm not a very smart person and mine always turn out oval. When I work with this, I always like to work on top of a silpat because it's naturally non-stick.

Fold the edges of the dough inward and form a small crust on the dough. If you have any scraps remaining, you can add it into the crust if you want. Bake the dough for 10 minutes. Just enough so they're starting to get slightly golden brown. Remove the crust from the oven and let cool for a moment. Slice a medium vine tomato and put half on each pizza along with 2 tbsp. Rao's tomato sauce per pizza. Aww...they look like little peace signs. Top these suckers with cheese – about 2 oz. Shredded Cheddar per pizza. Chop up the bell peppers. You can use 1 bell pepper or 2 different colors. I am using 1/3 red bell pepper and 1/3 yellow bell pepper for the topping. Arrange the peppers how you like and throw it back in the oven for another 8-10 minutes. Remove the pizzas from the oven and let cool. In the meantime, slice up some fresh basil and have it ready for serving. Serve it up – top with fresh basil and enjoy the fresh bites of summer!

Nutrition Info

Calories 31.32g Fats

6.46g Net Carbs 22.26g Protein.

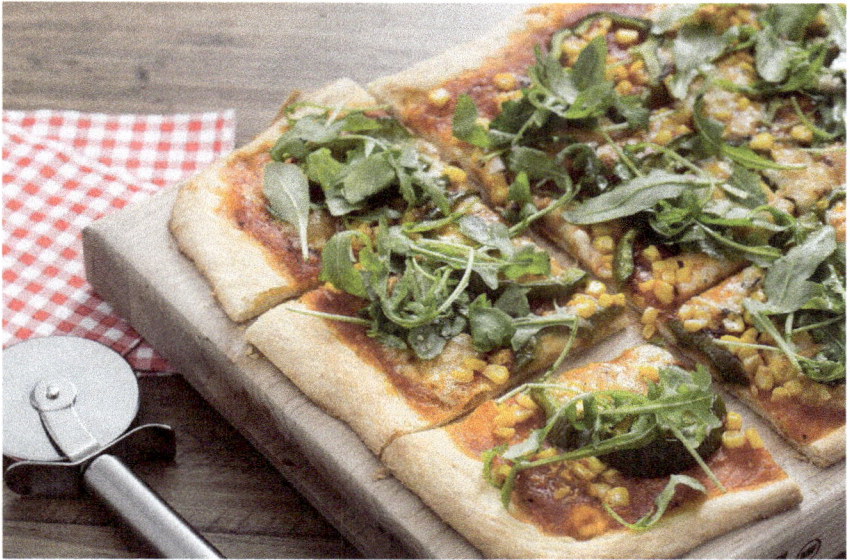

Keto Cheesy Broccoli & Cauliflower Rice

Creamy, delicious, and incredibly easy, this Keto Cheesy Broccoli & Cauliflower Rice makes the perfect low carb side dish!

Prep Time: 5 minutes Cook Time: 8 minutes Total Time: 13 minutes Servings: 4

Ingredients

3 cups riced cauliflower 1 cup riced broccoli

1 tablespoon butter

1/2 teaspoon kosher salt

1/4 teaspoon ground black pepper

1/4 teaspoon garlic powder pinch of ground nutmeg

1/2 cup shredded sharp cheddar cheese 1/4 cup mascarpone cheese

Instructions

Combine the cauliflower, broccoli, butter, salt, pepper, garlic powder, and nutmeg in a medium sized microwave safe bowl and microwave on high for 4 minutes. Stir.

Microwave for an additional 2 minutes. Stir.

Add the cheddar cheese and microwave an additional 2 minutes.

Remove from the microwave carefully and stir in the mascarpone cheese until creamy and fully incorporated.

Taste and adjust seasoning as desired. Serve hot.

Nutrition Info

Serving Size: 1 cup Calories: 138

Fat: 11g Carbohydrates: 5g Fiber: 3g

Protein: 6g

Low-Carb Vegetarian Greek Briam

Hands-on 30 minutes Total Time: 45 minutes

Ingredients (makes 6 servings)

1 small white or yellow onion, sliced (70 g/ 2.5 oz) 2 cloves garlic, minced

1/4 cup ghee (55 g/ 1.9 oz)

1 medium eggplant, diced (250 g/ 8.8 oz)

1/2 medium cauliflower, chopped (250 g/ 8.8 oz) 1/2 medium broccoli, chopped (150 g/ 3.5 oz)

1 medium green pepper, sliced (120 g/ 4.2 oz)

3 medium tomatoes, chopped (300 g/ 10.6 oz) 1/4 cup vegetable stock or water (60 ml/ 2 fl oz)

1   small zucchini, sliced (300 g/ 10.6 oz) 1/4 cup chopped parsley

1 tbsp chopped oregano or 1 tsp dried oregano 1/4 tsp salt, or to taste

freshly ground black pepper

1 1/2 cup crumbled feta cheese (225 g/ 8 oz) 1/2 cup extra virgin olive oil (120 ml/ 4 fl oz)

Instructions

Peel and slice the onion and crush the garlic. Place in a large casserole dish greased with ghee and cook over a medium-high heat for about 5 minutes or until fragrant and lightly browned. Low-Carb Vegetarian Greek Briam

Meanwhile, dice the eggplant into about 1/2-inch (1 cm) pieces. Once the onion & garlic are browned, add the eggplant. Cover with a lid, lower the heat to medium-low and cook for 3-5 minutes. Low-Carb Vegetarian Greek Briam

Meanwhile, cut the cauliflower and broccoli into small florets. Peel and slice the stalks. Low-Carb Vegetarian Greek Briam Add all to the casserole dish. Mix and keep cooking covered with a lid for 3-5 minutes. Slice the green pepper. Low-Carb Vegetarian Greek Briam

Roughly chop the tomatoes. Add both to the casserole dish, pour in vegetable stock or water, mix and cover with a lid. Cook for another 5 minutes. Low-Carb Vegetarian Greek Briam

Meanwhile, slice the zucchini. Add the slices to the dish and mix. Cover with a lid and cook for 5-10 minutes or until the zucchini is tender. Low-Carb Vegetarian Greek Briam

Add freshly chopped parsley and oregano, salt and pepper. Leave some parsley for garnish. Mix and top with crumbled feta cheese. Low-Carb Vegetarian Greek Briam

Place under a preheated broiler and cook for about 5 minutes or until the feta is lightly browned. Place on a cooling rack and leave to rest for 5 minutes. Finally, garnish with the reserved parsley and drizzle with olive oil. Low-Carb Vegetarian Greek

 Briam

Enjoy hot or cold. Serve full serving as a main dish, or half serving as a side. To store, refrigerate for up to 3 days.

Nutrition Info: Net carbs9.3 grams Protein8.7 grams Fat35.8 grams Calories 400 kcal

Cauliflower Confetti Kale Pecan Salad

Prep Time 15 minutes Total Time 15 minutes Servings 8

Ingredients

Instructions

1 small purple cauliflower or 2 cups or regular white cauliflower

1/2 cup red pepper chopped 1/2 cup yellow pepper chopped 1/2 cup chopped scallions

4 cups curly fresh kale stems removed 1/2 cup toasted chopped pecans

3 tbsp extra virgin olive oil 1/4 cup lemon juice

salt and pepper to taste

Optional: 2 ounces asiago cheese chunks

Remove stem and slice cauliflower very thinly.

Add cauliflower, peppers, scallions and kale to a serving bowl or dish.

Top with pecans.

Whisk oil and lemon juice together. Season with salt and pepper to taste. Toss dressing in bowl.

Refrigerate until ready to serve.

Serve as a side dish or add some protein for a main meal.

Nutrition Info

Calories 112 Calories from Fat 83 Fat 9.2g

Saturated Fat 1.1g Sodium 59mg Carbohydrates 7.6g Fiber 2.1g

Sugar 1.3g Protein 2.3g

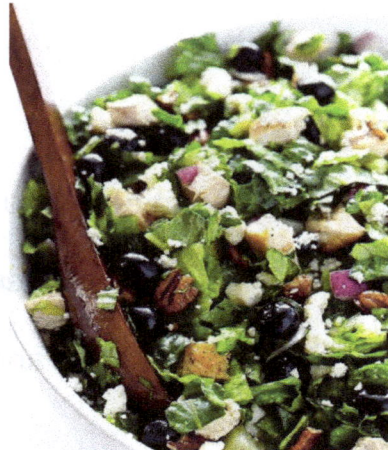

Roasted Mushroom and Walnut Cauliflower Grits

Servingss 4

Ingredients

6 ounces baby portobello mushrooms, sliced

3 cloves garlic, minced

1 tablespoon rosemary

½ cup walnuts, chopped

1 tablespoon smoked paprika

2 tablespoons olive oil

588 g cauliflower, 1 medium head

½ cup water

1 cup half and half

1 cup shredded sharp cheddar

2 tablespoons butter

Salt to taste

Instructions

Heat oven to 400°F and line a cookie sheet with foil. Combine the sliced mushrooms, minced garlic, rosemary, walnuts, and smoked paprika in a small dish and drizzle with olive oil. Toss to coat and season with salt. Spread the mixture evenly on the cookie sheet and roast in the oven for 15 minutes.

Process one head of cauliflower florets in a food processor by pulsing until very fine.

Steam the processed cauliflower in a medium pot, covered, with ½ cup water for 5 minutes or until the mixture is slightly tender. You don't want it to be too soft since it will need to resemble grits.

Pour half and half into the cauliflower grits, stir and simmer on medium-low heat for 3 minutes. This is just enough time to heat the milk.

Stir in the sharp cheddar and butter and reduce heat to low until the mixture is creamy and well combined. Season with salt to taste. If you like your grits runny add another ¼ c. water.

Remove roasting pan from the oven once your mushrooms are soft and the edges are a deep brown.

Serve the cauliflower grits hot, topped with the mushroom mixture and extra butter if desired!

Nutrition Info

455 Calories 36.5g Fats 11.28g Net Carbs 15.28g Protein.

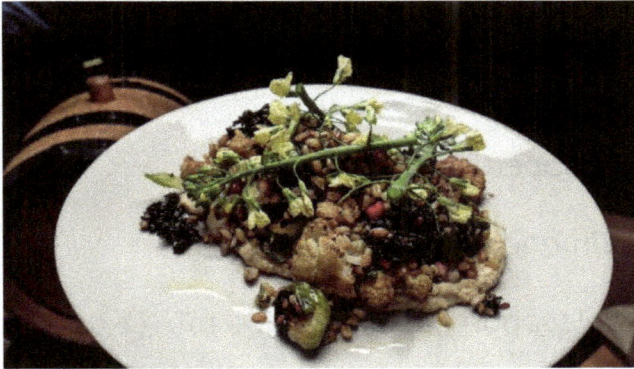

Mexican cauliflower patties

These low-carb Mexican cauliflower patties are everything! They are gluten- free and vegetarian, and will disappear in a flash, they taste THAT good.

Prep Time: 15 minutes Cook Time: 10 minutes Total Time: 50 minutes Servings: 8

Ingredients

1   small head cauliflower, cored and chopped into large florets 3 scallions minced

2   eggs, beaten

¼ cup chopped cilantro

¼ cup almond flour

1   tablespoon Mexican spice mix (I used this one) 1/4 teaspoon salt, plus coarse kosher salt to serve 1 cup shredded sharp cheddar cheese (4 oz)

2   tablespoons coconut oil lime wedges

Instructions

Bring 1 to 2 inches of water to a boil in a large saucepan fitted with a steamer basket. Preheat oven to 300ºF. Coat a baking sheet with cooking spray.

Add cauliflower to the steamer basket, cover and steam until the cauliflower is tender, 5 to 8 minutes. Remove basket from saucepan and allow to cool 10 minutes.

Meanwhile, stir scallions, eggs, cilantro, almond flour, spice mix and salt in a medium bowl.

Puree the cauliflower in a food processor fitted with a steel blade attachment until the cauliflower is paste-like, and becomes a little moist. It will not be completely smooth, more like tiny grains of rice. Add the cauliflower to the spice mixture and stir to combine. Add the cheddar and mix in evenly.

Heat 1 tablespoon oil in a large non-stick or cast iron skillet over medium heat. Mound scant ¼ cup portions of the cauliflower mixture into the oil. Cover with a lid and cook, adjusting heat to prevent scorching if necessary, until the cauliflower patties are set up and the bottoms are browned, 5 to 7 minutes. (If the patties seem like they will break apart they are not ready to flip.) Carefully flip the patties over and continue cooking until the second side is browned, and the patties are cooked through. Transfer the patties to the baking sheet and transfer to the oven to keep warm.

Repeat with the remaining 1 tablespoon oil and 4 portions of remaing cauliflower mixture, adjusting the heat if necessary. Serve with lime wedges and kosher salt.

Nutrition Info

Calories: 266

Sugar: 4 g

Sodium: 393 mg

Fat: 22 g

Saturated Fat: 13 g Carbohydrates: 7 g

Fiber: 1 g

Protein: 15 g

Mediterranean "Pasta"

Servings: Makes 4 Servings

Ingredients

2 large zucchini, spiral sliced (here is the spiral slicer I use) 1 cup spinach, packed

2 tbsp olive oil 2 tbsp butter

5 cloves garlic, minced

sea salt and black pepper, to taste

¼ cup sun-dried tomatoes 2 tbsp capers

2 tbsp Italian flat leaf parsley, chopped 10 kalamata olives, halved

¼ cup Parmesan cheese, shredded

¼ cup feta cheese, crumbled

Instructions

In a large sauté pan, over medium heat, add zucchini, spinach, olive oil, butter, garlic, sea salt and black pepper. Sauté until zucchini is tender and spinach is wilted. Drain excess liquid.

To the pan, add sun-dried tomatoes, capers, parsley, and kalamata olives. Mix in and sauté 2-3 minutes.

Remove from heat and toss with Parmesan and feta cheeses before serving.

Nutrition Info

Calories: 231 Fat: 20g Protein: 6.5g Net Carbs: 6.5g

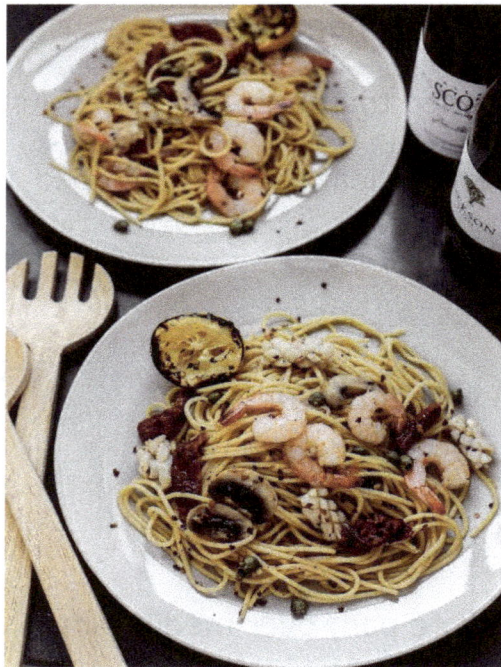

Grilled Halloumi Bruschetta

This low carb grilled halloumi makes a great side dish for your next cookout. Plus some great ideas for hosting the perfect backyard get together.

Prep Time 10 mins Cook Time 10 mins Total Time 20 mins Servings: 12 slices

Ingredients

2 medium tomatoes chopped 1/4 cup chopped fresh basil 2 to 3 cloves garlic minced 2 tbsp olive oil

Salt and pepper to taste

2 7- ounce packages Halloumi cheese (Cyprus grilling cheese)

Instructions

In a large, combine tomatoes, basil, garlic, olive oil, salt and pepper. Mix well and refrigerate (the flavours meld together well, so you can make this a few hours ahead).

Cut each piece of halloumi once crosswise and then cut into even 1/2 inch to 1/2-inch thin slices. You will get about 12 slices of cheese. Grill over medium heat until grill marks appear on the cheese, about 2 to 3 minutes per side. You will need to loosen the cheese with a metal spatula to turn.

Transfer to a serving platter and top with tomato basil mixture.

Nutrition Info

Calories 134

Calories from Fat 101 Fat 11.24g Cholesterol 25mg Carbohydrates 0.96g Fiber 0.26g

Protein 7.24g

Zucchini Ricotta Tart

Light and crispy puff pastry smeared with creamy herby ricotta and topped with fresh zucchini slices. Light and satisfying!

3 -4 servings

Ingredients

1   medium zucchini

2   teaspoons salt plus 1/8 teaspoon 1 tablespoon olive oil

½ cup 130gr ricotta cheese 1 handful parsley leaves

2 teaspoons lemon juice

1 Puff pastry sheet thawed

¼ teaspoon ground black pepper

1 egg yolk

Instructions

Cut the ends of the zucchini. Cut it lengthwise half way through (see photo above). And then thinly slice the zucchini. Place them in a colander and gently toss with 2 teaspoons of salt. Let it sit for about 30 minutes. This method sweats the zucchini and helps to get rid of excess water. Now, gently squeeze the zucchini slices between your palms in small batches and place them in a medium bowl. Drizzle with olive oil and set aside.

While the zucchini is sweating, place the ricotta, parsley, lemon juice and 1/8 teaspoon of salt in a food processor. Pulse until nice and smooth and the mixture is light green.

Preheat the oven to 400°F (200°C).

Unfold the puff pastry on a baking sheet lined with parchment paper. With a sharp knife, score the pastry about ¼ inch from the edges to create a border. Be careful not to cut all the way through though.

Spread the ricotta mixture evenly on the crust inside the border. Arrange the zucchini slices on the crust twisting each slice for a beautiful presentation. (If desired, simply lay the zucchini slices overlapping halfway.) Sprinkle some ground black pepper all over.

In a small dish, mix the egg yolk with 1 tablespoon of water to make an egg wash. Brush the egg wash on the edges of the tart. Bake the tart for 20-25 minutes, or until the crust is puffed up and golden brown. Cool on wire rack for 5-10 minutes before serving.

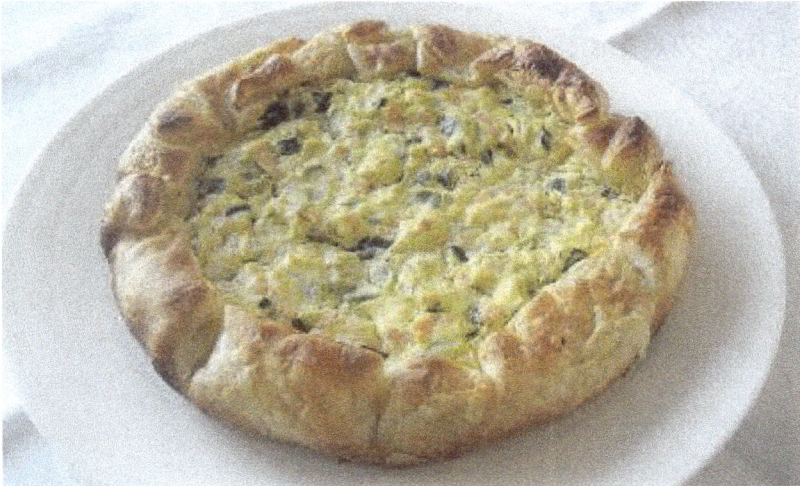

Soups and Salads

Cucumber, Mango, and Barley Salad

(Prep time: 5 min| Cooking Time: 20 min | serve: 2)

Ingredients

½ cup barley

¼ teaspoon ground cumin

½ cup water

½ mango, peeled and diced

½ cucumber, seeded and diced

½ red bell pepper, seeded and diced

½ cup broccoli

½ tablespoon chopped parsley

½ lime, juiced

Salt and ground black pepper to taste

Instructions

Put barley, water, and broccoli in Instant Pot. Lock the lid into place. Select Pressure Cook or Manual, and adjust the pressure to High and the time to 15 minutes. Make sure the vent on top is set to Sealing. After cooking, naturally, release the pressure. Unlock and remove the lid. Drain the beans and let cool for about 5 minutes. Mix mango, cucumbers, red bell peppers, chopped parsley, lime juice, salt, and black pepper in a bowl; stir in barley mixture. Serve immediately or chill in the refrigerator before serving.

Nutrition Facts

Calories 266, Total Fat 1.7g, Saturated Fat 0.3g, Cholesterol 0mg, Sodium 19mg, Total Carbohydrate 54.8g, Dietary Fiber 11.2g, Total Sugars 15.3g, Protein 8.1g

Greek Green Bean Salad with Feta and Tomatoes
(Prep time: 10 min| Cooking Time: 5 min | serve: 2)

Ingredients

1 cup fresh green beans, trimmed

2 tomatoes, chopped

1 tablespoon avocado oil

2 tablespoons vinegar

Salt and freshly ground black pepper to taste

1 onion, minced

¼ cup chopped fresh basil

1 teaspoon garlic powder

½ cup crumbled parmesan cheese

1 cup water

Instructions

Place the green beans in a steamer basket. Add 1 cup of water to the Instant Pot and place the steamer basket inside. Lock the lid into place. Select Steam and adjust the pressure to High and the time to 10 minutes. Pressure release naturally for 2 minutes, then quickly release any remaining pressure.

Combine green beans and tomatoes in a large bowl.

Stir together avocado oil, vinegar, salt, and pepper in a small bowl. Add onions, basil, and garlic powder.

Pour dressing over green beans and tomatoes and mix. Mix crumbled

parmesan cheese. Allow sitting for 20 minutes before serving.

Nutrition Facts

Calories 109, Total Fat 2.8g, Saturated Fat 1.2g, Cholesterol 5mg, Sodium 77mg, Total Carbohydrate

15.6g, Dietary Fiber 5g 18%, Total Sugars 6.7g, Protein 5.4g

Quick Edamame Salad

(Prep time: 10 min| Cooking Time: 5 min | serve: 2)

Ingredients

½ cup frozen shelled edamame

¼ cup sweet corn

¼ cup green peas

¼ cup black beans

½ red onion, minced

1 tablespoon coconut oil

½ teaspoon salt

½ teaspoon dried dill

¼ teaspoon ground black pepper

¼ teaspoon dried basil

¼ teaspoon garlic powder

1 cup water

Instructions

Place the edamame, sweet corn, black beans, peas in a steamer basket. Add 1 cup of water to the Instant Pot and place the steamer basket inside. Lock the lid into place. Select Steam and adjust the pressure to High and the time to 10 minutes. Pressure release naturally for 2 minutes, then quickly release any remaining pressure

Mix edamame, corn, peas, black beans, and red onion in a large bowl. Stir coconut oil, salt, dill, black pepper, basil, and garlic powder into an edamame mixture.

Chill in the refrigerator at least 30 minutes before serving.

Nutrition Facts

Calories 234, Total Fat 9g, Saturated Fat 6.3g, Cholesterol 0mg, Sodium 588mg, Total Carbohydrate

27.5g, Dietary Fiber 7.4g, Total Sugars 4.4g, Protein 10.8g

Green Bean and Potato Salad

(Prep time: 15 min| Cooking Time:15 min | serve: 2)

Ingredients

½ cup red potatoes

1 cup fresh green beans, trimmed and snapped

¼ cup chopped fresh basil

1 small red onion, chopped

Salt and pepper to taste

¼ cup balsamic vinegar

2 tablespoons Dijon mustard

2 tablespoons fresh lemon juice

1 teaspoon garlic powder

½ tablespoon coconut oil

Instructions

Place the potatoes in an Instant Pot, and fill with about 1-inch water. Lock the lid into place. Select Steam and adjust the pressure to High and the time to 10 minutes.

Pressure release naturally for 2 minutes, quickly release any remaining pressure, add green beans to the Instant Pot. Drain, calm, and cut potatoes into quarters. Transfer to a large bowl, and toss with fresh basil, red onion, salt, and pepper. Set aside. In a medium bowl, whisk together the balsamic vinegar, mustard, lemon juice, garlic powder, and coconut oil. Pour over the salad, and stir to coat. Taste and season with additional salt and pepper if needed.

Nutrition Facts

Calories 113, Total Fat 4.3g, Saturated Fat 3.1g, Cholesterol 0mg, Sodium 189mg, Total Carbohydrate 15.7g, Dietary Fiber 4g, Total Sugars 3.6g, Protein 3.2g

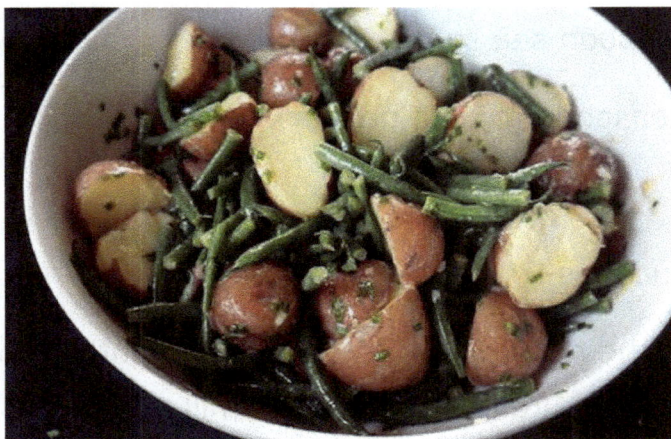

Lemon Millet Vegetable Salad

(Prep time: 10 min| Cooking Time: 5 min | serve: 2)

Ingredients

½ cup uncooked millet

1 cup water

½ carrot, chopped

1 cucumber, chopped

¼ cup walnuts

¼ cup pumpkin seeds

1 tablespoon olive oil

1 lemon, juiced

¼ teaspoon sea salt

1/8 teaspoon ground pepper

Instructions

Rinse the millet in a fine-mesh sieve until the water runs clear. Drain and place the millet in an Instant Pot. Add the water. Lock on the lid and set the Instant Pot to

1 minute cooking time at High Pressure. Make sure the vent on top is set to Sealing. Once the cooking time is up, let the pressure come down naturally for 10 minutes and release any remaining pressure.

Remove the lid and use a fork to fluff the millet. Add the carrots, cucumbers, walnuts, and pumpkin seeds to the millet and stir to combine. 6. Add the olive oil, lemon juice, salt, and pepper. Stir one more time to combine. Serve chilled or at room temperature.

Nutrition Facts

Calories 501, Total Fat 26.5g, Saturated Fat 3.5g, Cholesterol 0mg, Sodium 258mg, Total Carbohydrate 50.8g, Dietary Fiber 7.9g, Total Sugars 4.3g, Protein 14.9g

Crisp Green Bean Salad

(Prep time: 15 min| Cooking Time: 5 min | serve: 2)

Ingredients

1 cup fresh green beans, trimmed

1 tablespoon vinegar

½ teaspoon ginger powder

½ tablespoon toasted sesame seeds

1 teaspoon olive oil

½ teaspoon soy sauce

½ teaspoon garlic powder

1 tablespoon avocado oil

Salt and ground black pepper to taste

½ cup grape tomatoes

½ cup shredded carrot

½ cup zucchini, diced

1 cup water

Instructions

Place the green beans in a steamer basket. Add 1 cup of water to the Instant Pot and place the steamer basket inside. Lock the lid into place. Select Steam and adjust the pressure to High and the time to 10 minutes. Pressure release naturally for 2 minutes, then quickly release any remaining pressure. Combine vinegar, ginger powder, sesame seeds, olive oil, soy sauce, garlic powder in a bowl. Whisk avocado oil into the vinegar mixture until thoroughly incorporated; season with salt and black pepper. Toss green beans, grape tomatoes, and carrots, zucchini in a large bowl. Drizzle dressing over the green bean mixture; toss to coat.

Nutrition Facts

Calories 83, Total Fat 4.6g, Saturated Fat 0.7g, Cholesterol 0mg, Sodium 87mg, Total Carbohydrate

9.5g, Dietary Fiber 3.8g, Total Sugars 3.2g, Protein 2.8g

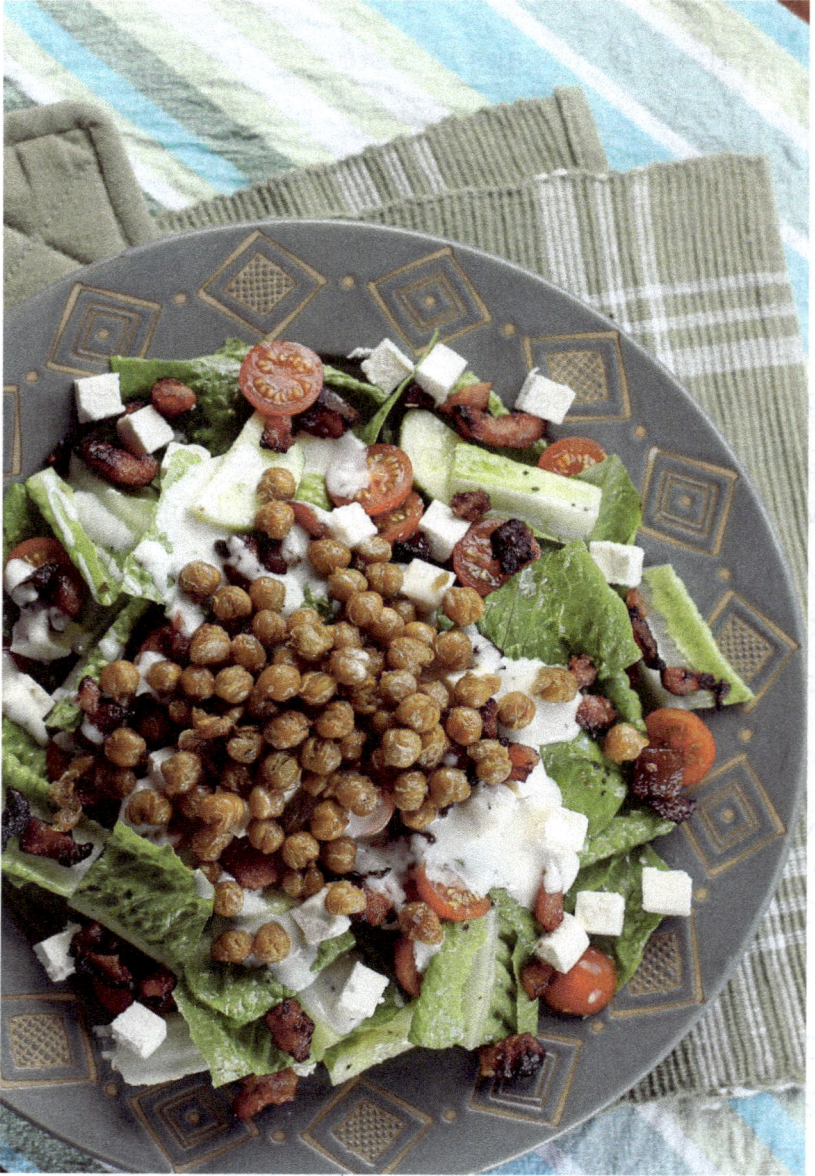

Broccoli and Noodle Salad

(Prep time: 15 min| Cooking Time: 5 min | serve: 2)

Ingredients

1 cup broccoli

½ cup noodles

1 bunch green onions, chopped

1 cup unsalted walnuts

1 cup sunflower seeds

½ cup honey

¼ cup olive oil

1 1/2 cups of water

Instructions

Pour 1 1/2 cups of water into the Instant Pot and insert the steam rack. Place noodles in a steamer basket and lower the steamer basket onto the steam rack. Secure the lid, making sure the vent is closed. Use the display panel and select the Manual or Pressure Cook function.

Use the + /- keys and program the Instant Pot for 5 minutes.

Whisk together the honey, olive oil. Pour over noodles and broccoli and toss to coat evenly. Refrigerate until chilled; top with walnuts and sunflower seeds before serving.

Nutrition Facts

Calories 560, Total Fat 46.4g, Saturated Fat 5.3g, Cholesterol 12mg, Sodium 22mg, Total Carbohydrate 24.3g, Dietary Fiber 4.9g, Total Sugars 6.3g, Protein 11.5g

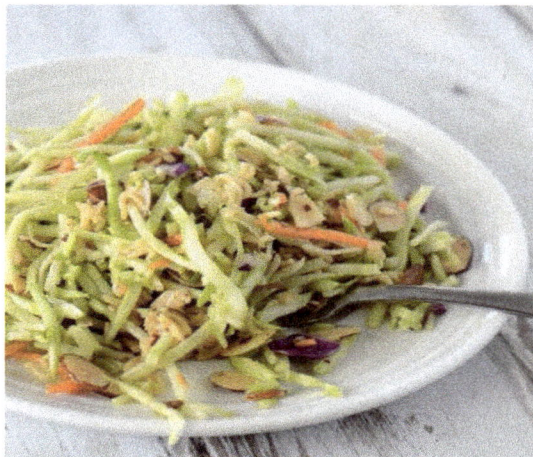

Greek Lentil Salad

(Prep time: 15 min| Cooking Time: 15 min | serve: 2)

Ingredients

1 cup brown lentils

½ cup crumbled goat cheese

1 cucumber, peeled and diced

1 tomato, diced

1small red onion, diced

2 cups water

1 lime juice

Salt and pepper to taste

Instructions

Pour the water into the Instant Pot and add the brown lentils. Lock the lid into place. Select Pressure Cook or Manual, and adjust the pressure to High and the time to 10 minutes. Make sure the vent on top is set to Sealing.

After cooking, naturally, release the pressure. Unlock and remove the lid. Drain the beans and let cool for about 5 minutes.

In a large bowl, combine the brown lentils, onions, cucumbers, tomatoes, lime juice, goat cheese, salt, and pepper. Toss, and chill until serving.

Nutrition Facts

Calories 112, Total Fat 3g, Saturated Fat 1.9g, Cholesterol 7mg, Sodium 108mg, Total Carbohydrate 15g, Dietary Fiber 3.9g, Total Sugars 5.5g, Protein 6.3g

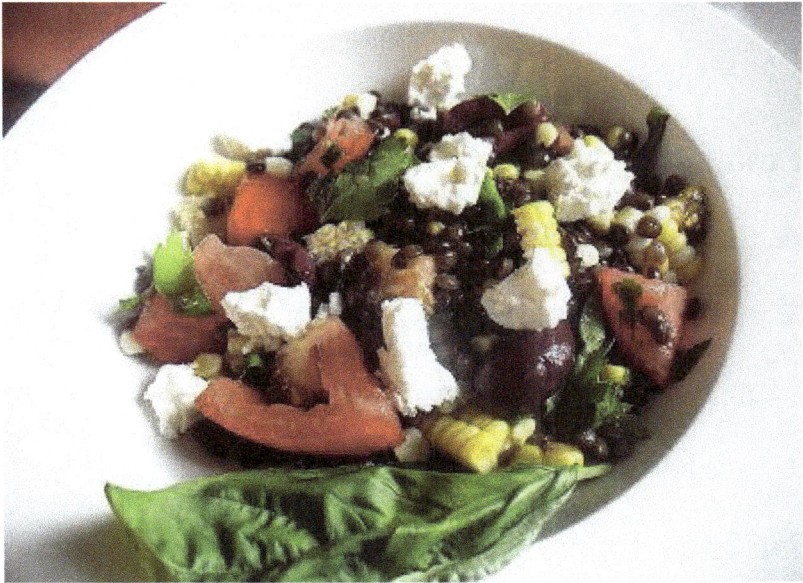

Red Quinoa and Avocado Salad

(Prep time: 15 min| Cooking Time: 15 min | serve: 2)

Ingredients

½ cup red quinoa

1 1/2 cups water

1 tomato, halved

½ cup diced cucumber

¼ cup diced red onion

1 tablespoon lime juice

½ teaspoon cumin seed

Salt and pepper to taste

2 cups kale leaves

1 avocado, peeled, pitted, and sliced

Instructions

Pour the quinoa into the Instant Pot. Add the water and kosher salt. Lock the lid into place. Select Pressure

Cook or Manual, and adjust the pressure to High and the time to 10 minutes. After cooking, let the pressure release naturally for 2 minutes, then quickly release any remaining pressure. Unlock the lid. Remove the pot from the base. Fluff the quinoa with a fork and let it cool for a few minutes. Transfer it to a medium bowl.

Once the quinoa has chilled, gently stir in the tomatoes, cucumber, and onion. Season with lime juice, cumin seed, salt, and pepper; stir to combine. Divide the kale onto salad plates, and top with the quinoa salad. Garnish with the avocado slices to serve.

Nutrition Facts

Calories 283, Total Fat 20.3g, Saturated Fat 4.2g, Cholesterol 0mg, Sodium 37mg, Total Carbohydrate

24.1g, Dietary Fiber 9.6g, Total Sugars 3.1g, Protein 4.8g

Dinner

Baked Crimini Mushrooms and Red Potatoes

Ingredients

1 pound red potatoes, halved

2 tablespoons extra virgin olive oil

1/2 pound Cremini mushrooms

8 cloves unpeeled garlic

2 tablespoons chopped fresh thyme

1 tablespoon extra-virgin olive oil, sea salt, and ground black pepper to taste

1/4 pound cherry tomatoes

3 tablespoons toasted pine nuts

1/4 pound spinach, thinly sliced

Directions:

Preheat your oven to 425 degrees F. Spread the potatoes in a pan Drizzle with 2 tablespoons of olive oil and roast for 15 minutes, turning once. Add the mushrooms with the stem sides up. Add the garlic cloves to the pan and cook until lightly browned. Sprinkle with thyme. Drizzle with 1 tablespoon olive oil and season with sea salt and black pepper. Return to the oven and bake for 5 min. Add the cherry tomatoes to the pan. Return to oven and bake until mushrooms become softened, for 5 min. Sprinkle the pine nuts over the potatoes and mushrooms. Serve with spinach.

Baked Shitake Mushrooms and Kohlrabi

Ingredients

1 pound kohlrabi, halved

2 tablespoons extra virgin olive oil

1/2 pound shitake mushrooms

8 cloves unpeeled garlic

3 tablespoons sesame oil, sea salt, and ground black pepper to taste

1/4 pound cherry tomatoes

3 tablespoons toasted cashew nuts

1/4 pound spinach, thinly sliced

Directions:

Spread the potatoes in a pan Drizzle with 2 tablespoons of oil, and Preheat your oven to 425 degrees F. roast for 15 minutes, turning once. Add the mushrooms with the stem sides up. Add the garlic cloves to the pan and cook until lightly browned. Drizzle with 1 tablespoon sesame oil and season with sea salt and black pepper. Return to the oven and bake for 5 min. Add the cherry tomatoes to the pan. Return to oven and bake until mushrooms become softened, for 5 min. Sprinkle the cashew nuts over the kohlrabi and mushrooms. Serve with spinach.

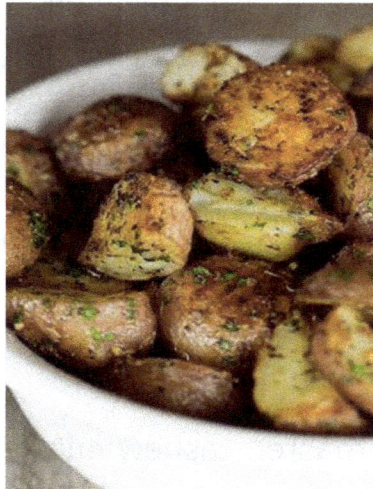

Baked Button Mushroom and Summer Squash

Ingredients

1 pound summer squash, halved

2 tablespoons extra virgin olive oil

1/2 pound button mushrooms

8 cloves unpeeled garlic

2 tsp. cumin 1 tsp. annatto seed

½ tsp. cayenne pepper

1 tablespoon extra-virgin olive oil

sea salt and ground black pepper to taste

1/4 pound cherry tomatoes

3 tablespoons toasted pine nuts

1/4 pound spinach, thinly sliced

Directions: Preheat, your oven to 425 degrees F.,
Spread the summer squash in a pan, Drizzle with 2
tablespoons of olive oil, and roast for 15 minutes,
turning once. Add the mushrooms with the stem sides

up. Add the garlic cloves to the pan and cook until lightly browned. Sprinkle with cumin, cayenne pepper, and annatto seeds. Drizzle with 1 tablespoon olive oil and season with sea salt and black pepper. Return to the oven and bake for 5 min. Add the cherry tomatoes to the pan. Return to oven and bake until mushrooms become softened, for 5 min. Sprinkle the pine nuts over the summer squash and mushrooms. Serve with spinach.

Baked Spinach and Butternut Squash

Ingredients

1 ½ pounds butternut squash, peeled and cut into 1-inch chunks

½ red onion, thinly sliced

¼ cup water

½ vegetable stock cube, crumbled

1 tbsp. extra virgin olive oil

½ tsp cumin

½ tsp annatto seeds

½ tsp cayenne pepper

½ tsp hot chili powder

Black pepper

½ pound fresh spinach, roughly chopped

Directions:

Put all of the ingredients in a slow cooker except the last one. Top with handfuls of spinach and stuff the slow cooker with it. If you can't fit it all in at once, let the first batch cook first and add some more spinach. Cook for 3or 4 hours on medium until squash becomes soft. Scrape the sides and serve.

Rutabagas Curry

(Prep time: 10 min |Cooking Time: 20 min | serve: 2)

Ingredients

4 rutabagas, peeled and cored from the top

1 tablespoon vegetable oil

½ onion, finely chopped

1 teaspoon ginger powder

1 teaspoon garlic powder

1 red tomato, pureed

¼ teaspoon turmeric

¼ tablespoon red chili powder

¼ teaspoon Garam masala

½ teaspoon salt

5 almonds

1/8 cup milk warm

½ tablespoon dried fenugreek leaves

Basil leaves

Instructions

Soak almonds in warm milk for 10 minutes and set aside. Set Instant Pot to Sauté mode. Once the —Hot‖ sign displays, add vegetable oil. Add onions and cook for 2 minutes with a glass lid on, stirring few times. Add ginger and garlic powder, cook for 30 seconds. Add the carved-out pieces from the rutabagas. Add tomato paste, turmeric, red chili powder, Garam masala, and salt. Cook everything on Sauté mode for 2 minutes with a glass lid on, stirring a couple of times. With a small spoon, carefully fill the rutabagas with the cooked masala/gravy and line them all in the Instant Pot insert. Add 1/2 cup of water. Close the Instant Pot, using the Manual function, set the cooker to High Pressure for 8 minutes. When time is up, quickly release the pressure.

Blend milk and almonds to make a smooth paste. Stir in dried fenugreek leaves, almond paste, and chopped basil.

Set Instant Pot to Sauté mode, mix everything. Add salt to taste. Bring to a gentle boil, and then turn Instant Pot off. Serve with hot and. Enjoy!

Nutrition Facts

Calories 219, Total Fat 9.4g, Saturated Fat 1.7g, Cholesterol 1mg, Sodium 664mg, Total Carbohydrate

31g, Dietary Fiber 9.3g, Total Sugars 18.7g, Protein 6.2g

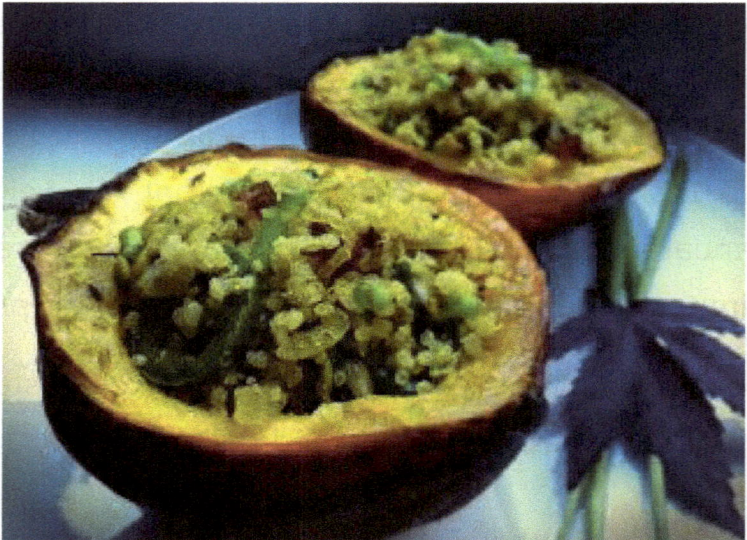

Baked Brussel Sprouts & Red Onion Glazed with Balsamic Vinegar

Ingredients

1 (16 ounces) package fresh Brussels sprouts

2 small red onions, thinly sliced

¼ cup and 1 tbsp. extra-virgin olive oil, divided

1/4 teaspoon sea salt

1/4 teaspoon rainbow peppercorns

1 shallot, chopped

1/4 cup balsamic vinegar

1 tablespoon chopped fresh rosemary

Directions:

Preheat your oven to 425 degrees F (220 degrees C). Grease a baking pan.

Combine Brussels sprouts and onion in a bowl. Add 4 tablespoons of olive oil, salt, and peppercorns. Toss to coat and spread the sprout mixture on the pan. Bake in the oven until sprouts and red onion becomes tender, for about 25 to 30 minutes. Heat the remaining tablespoon of olive oil in a small skillet over medium-high heat Sauté the shallots until tender, for about 5 minutes. Add balsamic vinegar and cook until the glaze is reduced for about 5 minutes. Add rosemary into the balsamic glaze and pour over the sprouts.

Baked Purple Cabbage with Rainbow Peppercorns

Ingredients

1 (16 ounces) package fresh purple cabbage

2 small red onions, thinly sliced

1/2 cup and 1 tbsp. extra-virgin olive oil, divided

1/4 teaspoon sea salt

1/4 teaspoon rainbow peppercorns

1 shallot, chopped

1/4 cup balsamic vinegar

1 tsp. herbs de Provence

Directions:

Preheat your oven to 425 degrees F (220 degrees C). Grease a baking pan. Combine cabbage and onion in a bowl. Add 4 tablespoons of olive oil, salt, and peppercorns. Toss to coat and spread the sprouts mixture on the pan. Bake in the oven until sprouts and onion become tender, for about 25 to 30 minutes. Heat the remaining tablespoon of olive oil in a small skillet over medium-high heat Sauté the shallots until tender, for about 5 minutes. Add balsamic vinegar and cook until the glaze is reduced for about 5 minutes. Add herbs de Provence into the balsamic glaze and pour over the sprouts.

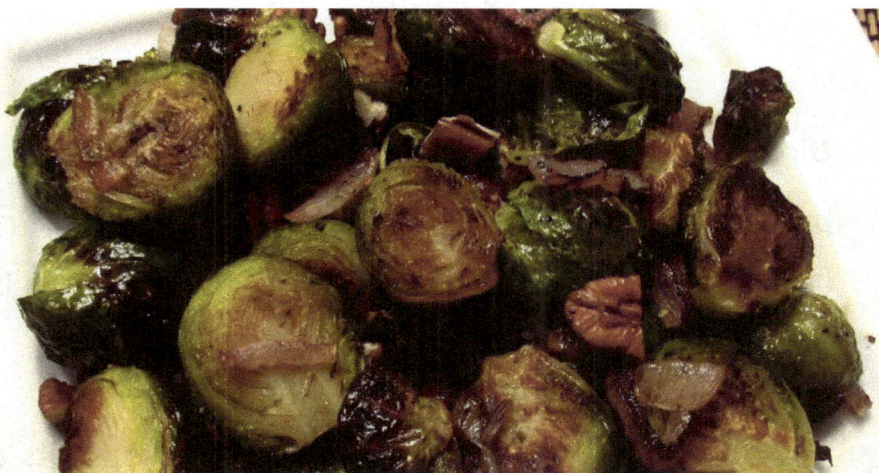

Roasted Savoy Cabbage and Vidalia Onion

Ingredients

1 (16 ounces) package fresh Savoy Cabbage

2 Vidalia onions, thinly sliced

¼ cup and 1 tbsp. extra-virgin olive oil, divided

1/4 teaspoon sea salt

1/4 teaspoon black peppercorns

shallot, chopped

1/4 cup white wine vinegar

1 tablespoon chopped fresh rosemary

Directions:

Preheat your oven to 425 degrees F (220 degrees C). Grease a baking pan. Combine cabbage and onion in a bowl. Add 4 tablespoons of olive oil, salt, and peppercorns. Toss to coat and spread the sprout mixture on the pan. Bake in the oven until sprouts and onion become tender, for about 25 to 30 minutes. Heat the remaining tablespoon of olive oil in a small skillet over medium-high heat Sauté the shallots until tender, for about 5 minutes. Add white wine vinegar and cook until the glaze is reduced for about 5 minutes. Add rosemary into the balsamic glaze and pour over the sprouts.

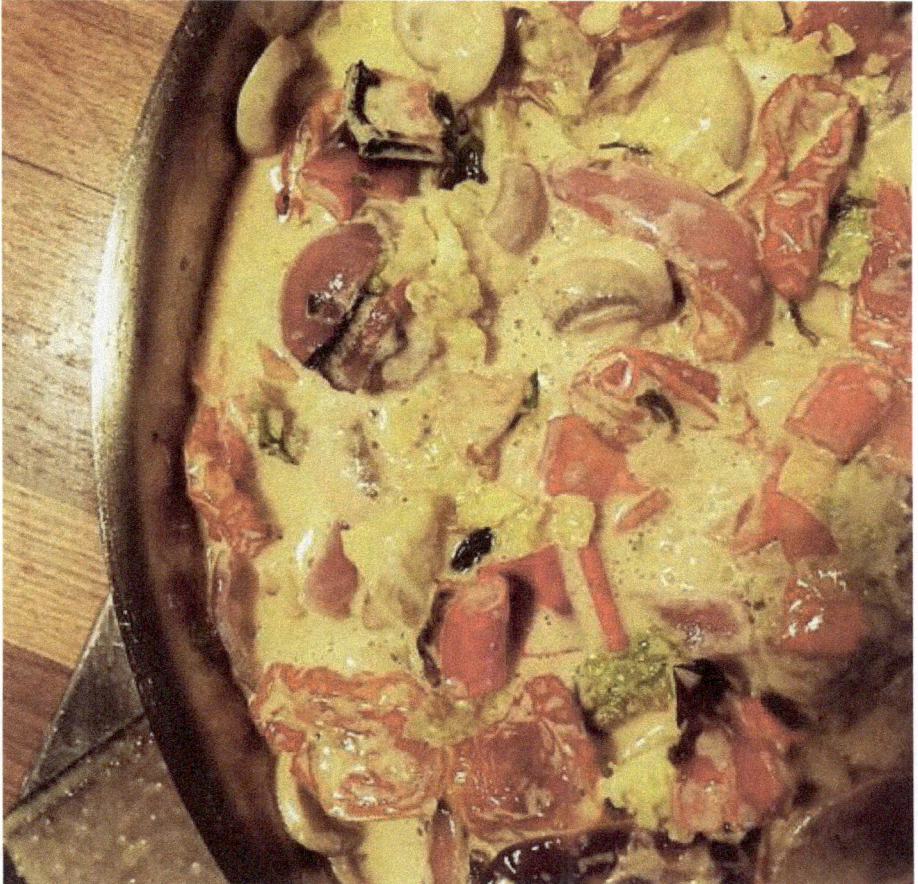

Baked Watercress and Summer Squash

Ingredients

1 ½ pounds summer squash, peeled and cut into 1-inch chunks

½ red onion, thinly sliced

¼ cup water

½ vegetable stock cube, crumbled

1 tbsp. sesame oil

½ tsp Chinese

5 spice powder

½ tsp Sichuan Peppercorns

½ tsp hot chili powder

Black pepper

½ pound fresh watercress, roughly chopped

Directions:

Put all of the ingredients in a slow cooker except the last one. Top with handfuls of watercress and stuff the slow cooker with it. If you can't fit it all in at once, let the first batch cook first and add some more watercress. Cook for 3 or 4 hours on medium until summer squash becomes soft. Scrape the sides and serve.

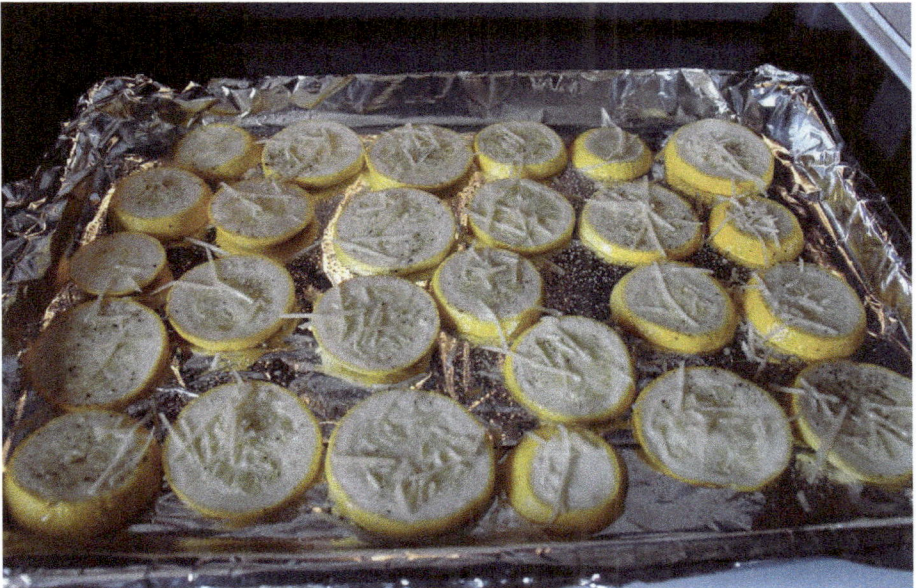

Curried Kale and Rutabaga

Ingredients

1 ½ pound Rutabaga, peeled and cut into 1-inch chunks

½ onion, thinly sliced

¼ cup water

½ vegetable stock cube, crumbled

1 tbsp. extra virgin olive oil

½ tsp cumin

½ tsp ground coriander

½ tsp garam masala

½ tsp hot chili powder Black pepper

½ pound fresh kale, roughly chopped

Directions:

Put all of the ingredients in a slow cooker except the last one. Top with handfuls of kale and stuff the slow cooker with it. If you can't fit it all in at once, let the first batch cook first and add some more kale. Cook for

3or 4 hours on medium until root vegetables become soft. Scrape the sides and serve.

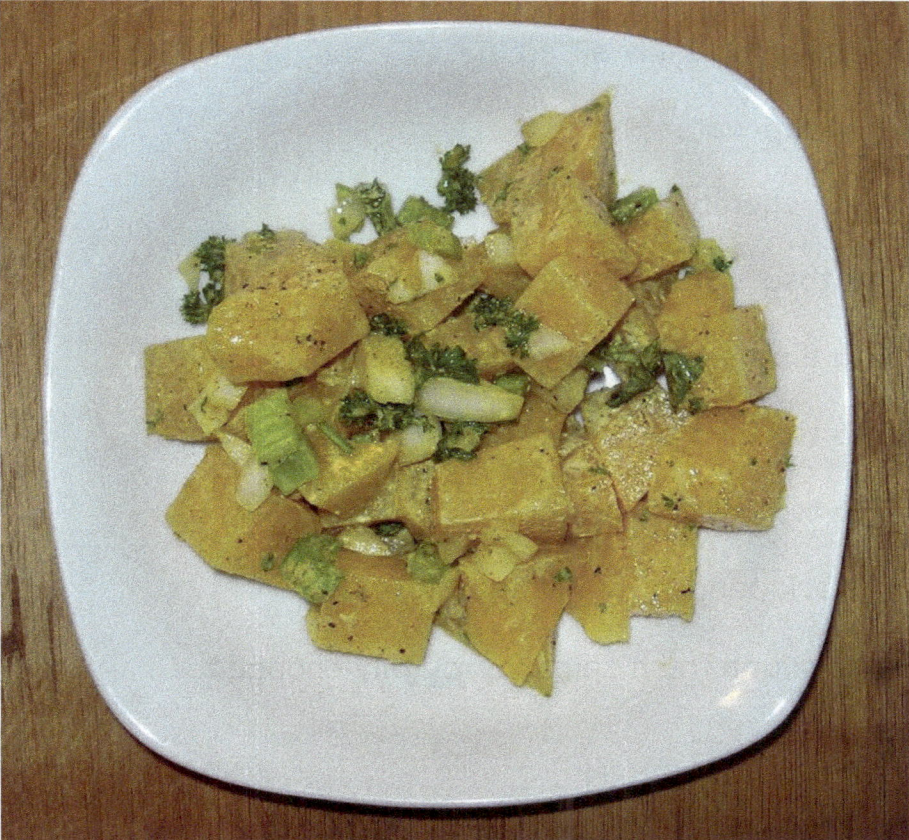

Buttered Potatoes and Spinach

Ingredients

1 ½ pounds red potatoes, peeled and cut into 1-inch chunks

½ onion, thinly sliced

¼ cup water

½ vegetable stock cube, crumbled

2 tbsp. salted butter

½ tsp herbs de Provence

½ tsp thyme

½ tsp hot chili powder

Black pepper

½ pound fresh spinach, roughly chopped

Directions:

Put all of the ingredients in a slow cooker except the last one. Top with handfuls of spinach and stuff the slow cooker with it. If you can't fit it all in at once, let the first batch cook first and add some more spinach. Cook

for 3or 4 hours on medium until potatoes become soft.
Scrape the sides and serve.

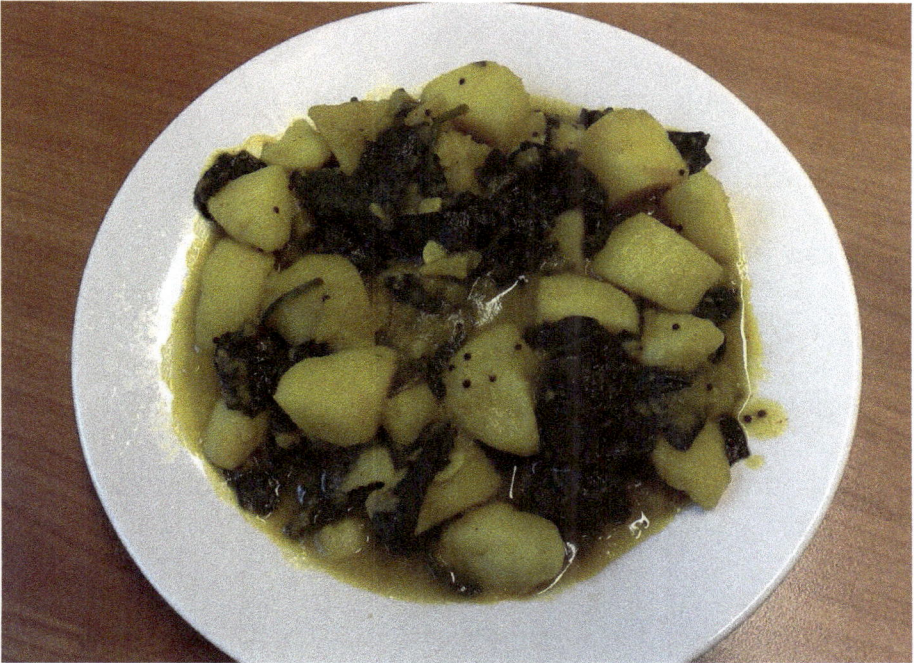

Roasted Vegan-Buttered Mustard Greens Carrots

Ingredients

1 ½ pounds carrots, peeled and cut into 1-inch chunks

½ onion, thinly sliced

¼ cup water

½ vegetable stock cube, crumbled

1 tbsp. butter

1 tsp garlic, minced

½ tsp lemon juice

Black pepper

½ pound fresh mustard greens, roughly chopped

Directions:

Put all of the ingredients in a slow cooker except the last one. Top with handfuls of mustard greens and stuff the slow cooker with it. If you can't fit it all in at once, let the first batch cook first and add some more mustard greens. Cook for 3or 4 hours on medium until carrots become soft. Scrape the sides and serve.

Smoky Roasted Swiss Chard and Cauliflower

Ingredients

1 ½ pounds cauliflower, peeled and cut into 1-inch chunks

½ red onion, thinly sliced

¼ cup water

½ vegetable stock cube, crumbled

1 tbsp. extra virgin olive oil

½ tsp cumin

½ tsp hot chili powder

Black pepper

½ pound fresh Swiss chard, roughly chopped

Directions:

Put all of the ingredients in a slow cooker except the last one. Top with handfuls of Swiss chard and stuff the slow cooker with it. If you can't fit it all in at once, let the first batch cook first and add some more Swiss chard. Cook for 3or 4 hours on medium until potatoes become soft. Scrape the sides and serve.

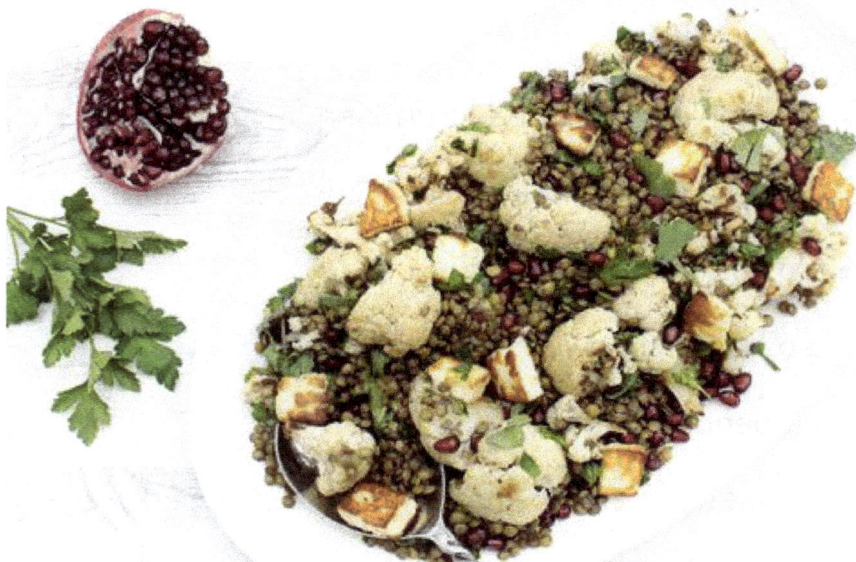

Sweets

Chocolate Chip Mini Muffins
Prep time: 5 min Cooking Time: 20 min serve: 2

Ingredients

½ cup coconut flour

1 egg

½ cup sugar-free chocolate chips

½ tablespoon vanilla extract

½ cup honey

1 tablespoon coconut

¼ teaspoon salt

¼ teaspoon baking soda

Instructions

Pour 1 cup of filtered water into the Instant Pot's inner pot, then insert the trivet. Using an electric mixer, combine coconut flour, egg, chocolate chips, vanilla, honey, coconut, salt, and baking soda. Mix thoroughly.

Using a sling if desired, place the pan onto the trivet and cover loosely with aluminium foil. Close the lid, set the Pressure Release to Sealing, and select Manual/Pressure Cook. Set the Instant Pot to 20 minutes on High Pressure and let cook.

Once cooked, let the pressure release naturally from the Instant Pot for about 10 minutes, then carefully switch the Pressure Release to Venting.

Open the Instant Pot and remove the pan. Let cool, serve and enjoy!

Nutrition Facts

Calories 366, Total Fat 4.8g, Saturated Fat 2.3g, Cholesterol 82mg , Sodium 508mg, Total Carbohydrate 76.8g, Dietary Fiber 1.7g , Total Sugars 70.6g, Protein 3.9g

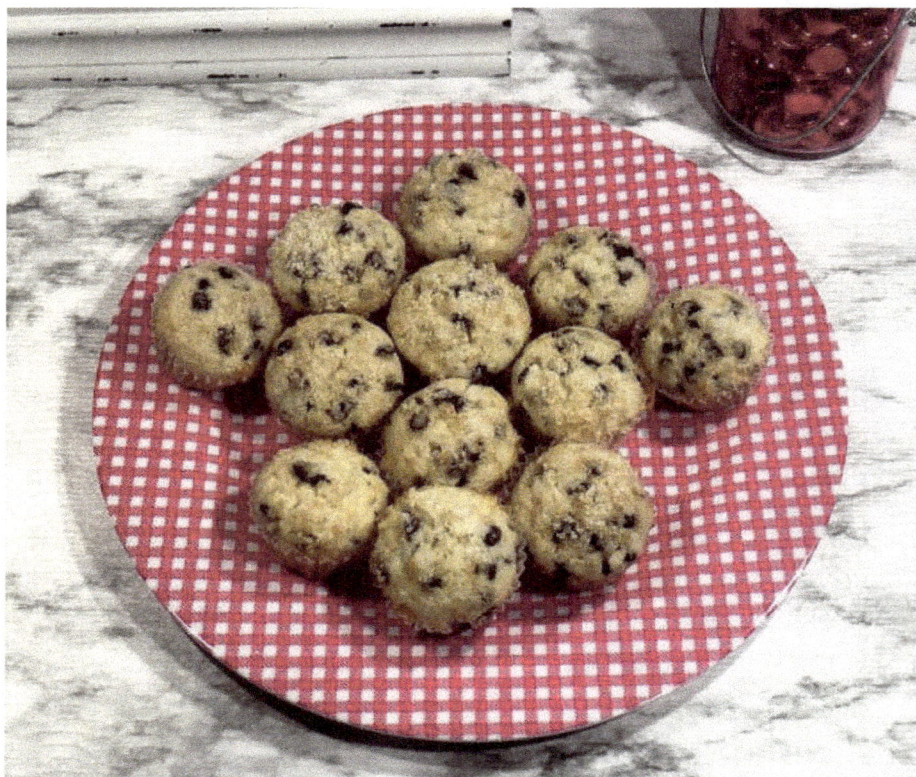

Pumpkin Spice Coffee Muffins

Prep time: 5 min Cooking Time: 20 min serve: 2

Ingredients

1/4 tablespoon coffee

1 cup coconut flour

2 tablespoons honey

½ cup pumpkin puree

1 tablespoon coconut oil

1 egg

1 teaspoon baking soda

¼ teaspoon ground allspice

½ teaspoon baking powder

1 tablespoon chocolate chips

Directions

In the instant pot's inner pot, put water then insert the trivet. Combine warm water and coffee in a cup until coffee is dissolved; pour into a large bowl. Mix coconut flour, honey, pumpkin puree, coconut oil, egg, baking soda, salt, allspice, and baking powder into coffee until batter is thoroughly mixed; fold in chocolate chips. Fill muffin cups with batter.

Using a sling if desired, place the pan onto the trivet and cover loosely with aluminium foil. Close the lid, set the Pressure Release to Sealing, and select Manual/Pressure

Cook. Set the Instant Pot to 20 minutes on High Pressure and let cook.

Once cooked, let the pressure release naturally from the Instant Pot for about 10 minutes, then carefully switch the Pressure Release to Venting.

Open the Instant Pot and remove the pan. Let cool, serve and enjoy!

Nutrition Facts

Calories 235, Total Fat 11.8g, Saturated Fat 8.8g, Cholesterol 83mg, Sodium 1266mg, Total Carbohydrate 30.3g, Dietary Fiber 4.6g , Total Sugars 22.6g, Protein 4.9g

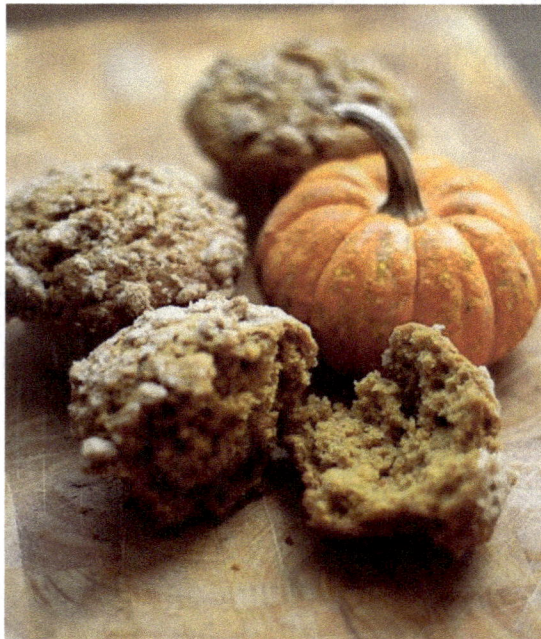

Blueberry Cream Muffins

Prep time: 10 min Cooking Time: 20 min serve: 2

Ingredients

1 egg

2 tablespoons maple syrup

1 tablespoon coconut oil

½ teaspoon vanilla extract

½ cup coconut flour

½ teaspoon salt

½ teaspoon baking soda

2 tablespoons coconut cream

2 tablespoons blueberries

Instructions

Grease 4 muffin cups or line with paper muffin liners. In large bowl beat egg, gradually add maple syrup while beating. Continue beating while slowly pouring in oil. Stir in vanilla. In a separate bowl, stir together flour, salt and baking soda.

Stir dry ingredients into egg mixture alternately with coconut cream. Gently fold in blueberries. Scoop batter into prepared muffin cups. Place the pan onto the trivet and cover loosely with aluminium foil. Close the lid, set the Pressure Release to Sealing, and select Manual/Pressure Cook. Set the Instant Pot to 20 minutes on High Pressure and let cook.

Once cooked, let the pressure release naturally from the Instant Pot for about 10 minutes, then carefully switch the Pressure Release to Venting.

Open the Instant Pot and remove the pan. Let cool, serve and enjoy!

Nutrition Facts

Calories 215, Total Fat 13.6g, Saturated Fat 10.7g, Cholesterol 82mg, Sodium 946mg, Total Carbohydrate 19.9g, Dietary Fiber 3.1g, Total Sugars 14.1g , Protein 4.2g

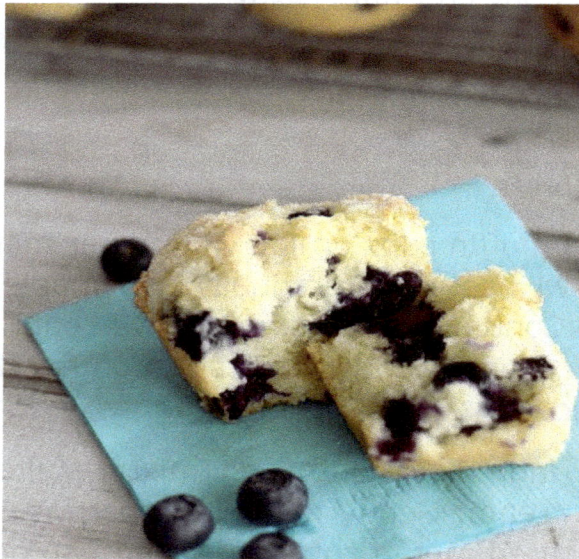

Apple Pumpkin Muffins

Prep time: 15 min Cooking Time: 20 min serve: 2

Ingredients

½ cup almond flour

¼ cup coconut flour

½ cup honey

¼ tablespoon pumpkin pie spice

¼ teaspoon baking soda

¼ teaspoon salt

1 egg

1 tablespoon pumpkin puree

½ tablespoon coconut oil

½ cup peeled and chopped apples

3 tablespoons butter, softened

½ tablespoon maple syrup

¼ cup wheat flour

1 teaspoon ground cinnamon

Instructions

 Combine coconut flour, almond flour, honey, pumpkin pie spice, baking soda, and salt in a large bowl. Mix egg, pumpkin, and coconut oil in a small bowl. Stir egg mixture into flour mixture until just moistened; fold in apples. Fill prepared muffin cups 2/3 full.

Combine butter, ½ cup maple syrup, ¼ cup whole wheat flour, and cinnamon in a small bowl; sprinkle over muffin batter.

Place the pan onto the trivet and cover loosely with aluminium foil. Close

the lid, set the Pressure Release to Sealing, and select Manual/Pressure Cook. Set the Instant Pot to 20 minutes on High Pressure and let cook.

Once cooked, let the pressure release naturally from the Instant Pot for about 10 minutes, then carefully switch the Pressure Release to Venting.

Open the Instant Pot and remove the pan. Let cool, serve and enjoy!

Nutrition Facts

Calories 383, Total Fat 18.7g, Saturated Fat 8g, Cholesterol 64mg , Sodium 308mg, Total Carbohydrate

48.2g, Dietary Fiber 3.2g , Total Sugars 37.7g, Protein 5.6g

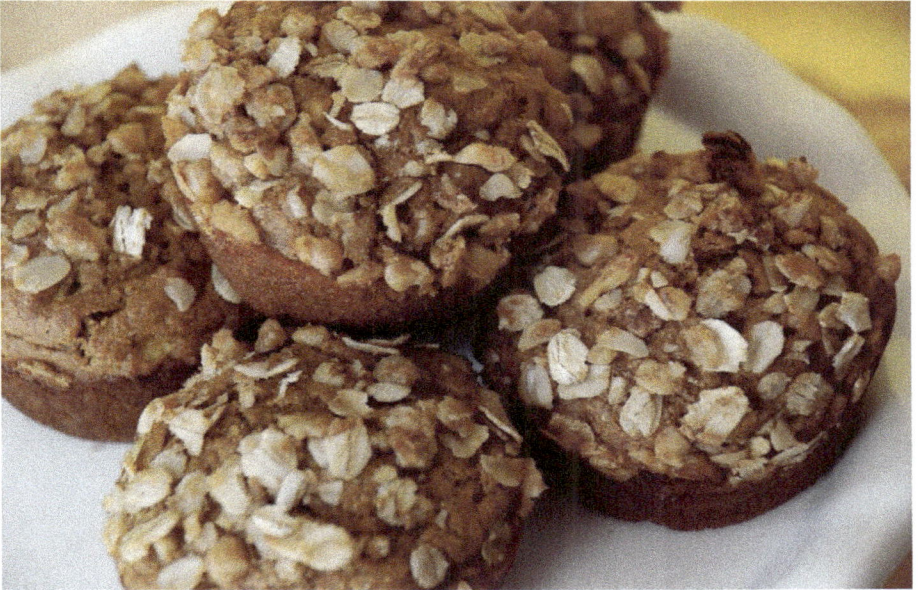

Pineapple Zucchini Muffins

Prep time: 30 min Cooking Time: 20 min serve: 2

Ingredients

½ cup coconut flour

½ tablespoon maple syrup

¼ teaspoon baking powder

½ teaspoon baking soda

½ teaspoon ground cinnamon

1tablespoon coconut oil

1 egg

3 tablespoons shredded zucchini

1 tablespoon crushed pineapple, drained

½ teaspoon vanilla extract

Instructions

In a large bowl, combine coconut flour, maple syrup, baking powder, baking soda, cinnamon and salt. Make a well in the centre, and pour in the oil, egg, zucchini, pineapple and vanilla. Mix until smooth. Fill muffin cups 2/3 to 3/4 packed.

Place the pan onto the trivet and cover loosely with aluminium foil. Close the lid, set the Pressure Release to Sealing, and select Manual/Pressure Cook. Set the Instant Pot to 20 minutes on High Pressure and let cook.

Once cooked, let the pressure release naturally from the Instant Pot for about 10 minutes, then carefully switch the Pressure Release to Venting.

Open the Instant Pot and remove the pan. Let cool, serve and enjoy!

Nutrition Facts

Calories 64, Total Fat 4.8g, Saturated Fat 3.5g, Cholesterol 41mg , Sodium 470mg, Total Carbohydrate 3.7g, Dietary Fiber 0.9g, Total Sugars 2.1g, Protein 1.7g

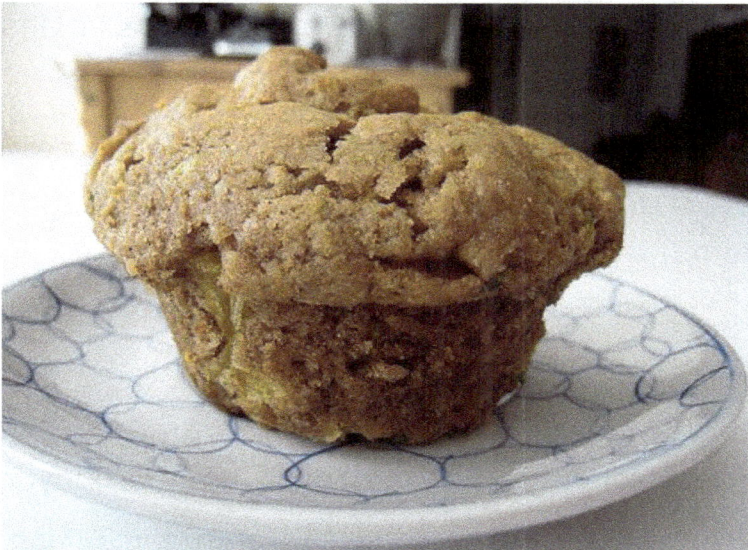

Blackberries Compote

Prep time: 15 min Cooking Time: 20 min serve: 2

Ingredients

4 cups fresh blackberries

¼ cup maple syrup

1 teaspoon freshly squeezed lemon juice

1 teaspoon orange juice

Instructions

Wash all the blackberries.

Add the blackberries and maple syrup to the Instant Pot. Add the lemon juice and orange juice

Lock the lid in place. Select Pressure Cook or Manual, and adjust the pressure to High and the time to 2 minutes. After cooking, let the pressure release naturally for 10 minutes, then quickly release any remaining pressure.

Unlock the lid. Taste the berries (carefully—they're hot) and adjust the sweetness if necessary.

Nutrition Facts

Calories 250, Total Fat 1.5g, Saturated Fat 0.1g, Cholesterol 0mg , Sodium 7mg, Total Carbohydrate

54.4g, Dietary Fiber 15.3g , Total Sugars 37.5g, Protein 4g

Raspberry-Vanilla Barley Pudding

Prep time: 10 min Cooking Time: 45 min serve: 2

Ingredients

1 cup water

1 cup coconut milk

1 tablespoon honey

½ cup raspberries fresh

½ cup barley

¼ teaspoon nutmeg

¼ teaspoon vanilla

½ cup coconut cream

Instructions

Select Sauté on the Instant Pot and adjust to normal. Add the coconut milk, water, honey, to the pot.

Press cancel. Stir in the barley and nutmeg and vanilla into the pot. Secure the lid on the Instant Pot.

Close the pressure-release valve. Select porridge. When cooking is complete, use a natural-release to depressurize.

Remove and Stir in fresh raspberries and cream.

Nutrition Facts

Calories 502,Total Fat 29.9g, Saturated Fat 25.7g, Cholesterol 0mg , Sodium 28mg, Total Carbohydrate

49.3g, Dietary Fiber 10.7g, Total Sugars 13.2g, Protein 8.5g

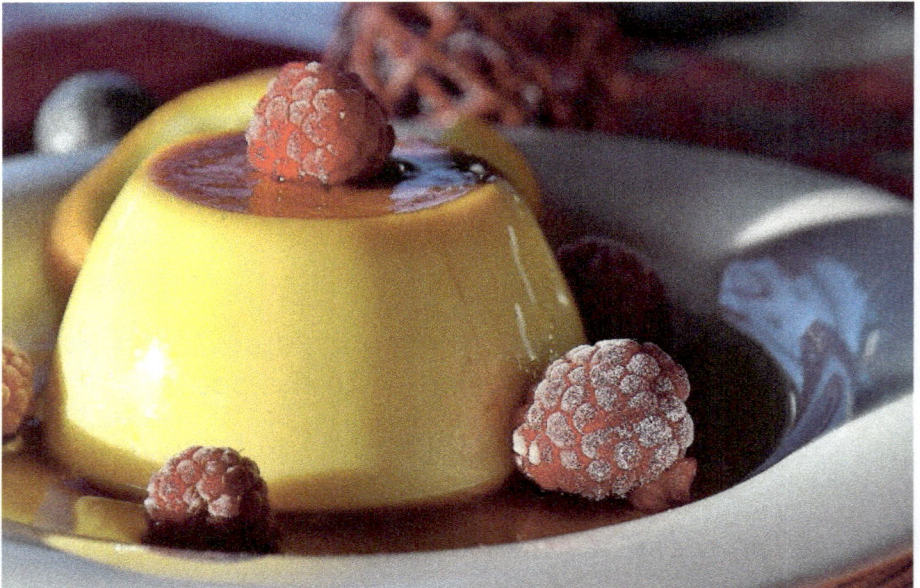

Nectarines Cobbler

Prep time: 10 min Cooking Time: 20 min serve: 2

Ingredients

4 fresh Nectarines, sliced

1 tablespoon honey

½ tablespoon coconut flour

1 tablespoon corn-starch

½ teaspoon lemon juice

1/2 cup Water

For the Topping

½ cup coconut flour

1 tablespoon honey

½ teaspoon baking powder

¼ teaspoon salt

2 tablespoon butter

¼ cup buttermilk

Instructions

Combine Nectarines, honey, coconut flour, corn-starch, lemon juice. Pour ½ cup water in the bottom of the Instant Pot, turn it on to Sauté, and boil the water. Add the Nectarines and let it cook.

In the meantime, for the topping, mix the coconut flour, honey, baking powder, and salt. Cut in the butter with a pastry cutter until pea size. Stir in the buttermilk.

Drop spoonful of the topping onto the Nectarines mixture, close the lid, select manual pressure high and set the time for 20 minutes. Natural pressure release and serve. Best served with vanilla ice cream.

Nutrition Facts

Calories 228, Total Fat 7.7g, Saturated Fat 5g, Cholesterol 16mg , Sodium 210mg, Total Carbohydrate 34.6g, Dietary Fiber 8.7g, Total Sugars 17.2g, Protein 3.8g

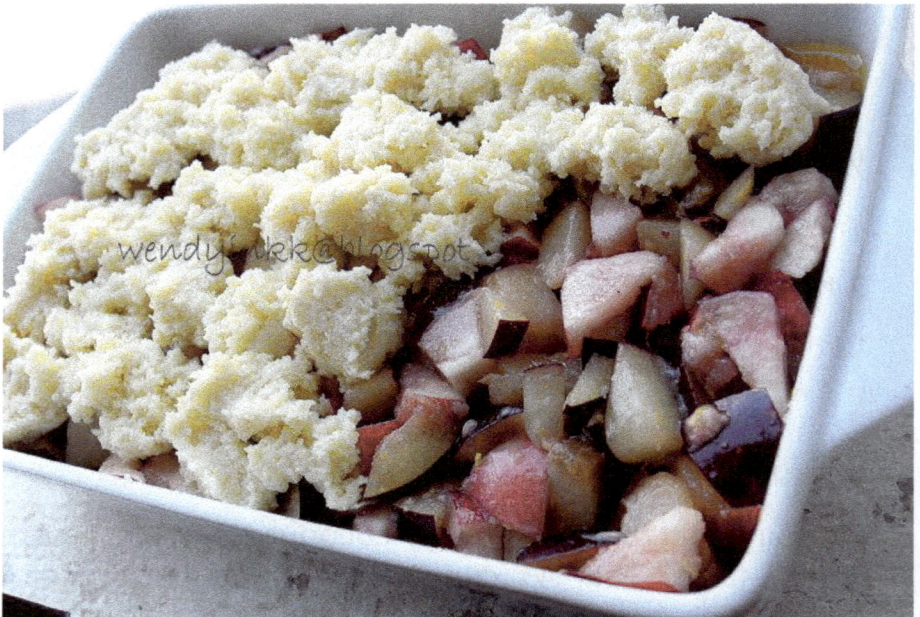

Hazelnuts Corn Syrup Mousse

Prep time: 15 min Cooking Time: 25 min serve: 2

Ingredients

½ tablespoon butter melted

1 egg

½ cup heavy cream

¼ cup corn syrup

1 cup hazelnuts

Chocolate Ganache topping optional

Directions

Using a paper towel, coat the inside of a spring form cake pan or oven proof casserole pan with coconut oil.

Line the bottom and sides of the pan with parchment paper and set aside.

Put the egg, heavy cream, and corn syrup into a blender and mix, scraping down the sides as needed, until completely smooth. Pour the mixture into the pan.

Pour 1 cup of water into the Instant Pot and place the trivet inside. Place the pan on top of the trivet and close the lid tightly.

Press Manual and adjust time to 25 minutes pressure cooking. When the timer ends, let pressure naturally release.

Open the lid and carefully lift out the trivet and place the pan on a cooling rack for 30-45 minutes.

When cooled, invert the pan onto a platter, carefully lift the parchment paper from the side.

Invert it again onto another platter, loosely cover and refrigerate overnight.

If you are using chocolate ganache topping, you can make it before serving, let it cool a little and cover the Hazelnuts Mousse and serve immediately.

Nutrition Facts

Calories 504, Total Fat 36.1g, Saturated Fat 9.3g, Cholesterol 123mg , Sodium 43mg, Total Carbohydrate 36.7g, Dietary Fiber 3.6g , Total Sugars 12g, Protein 9g

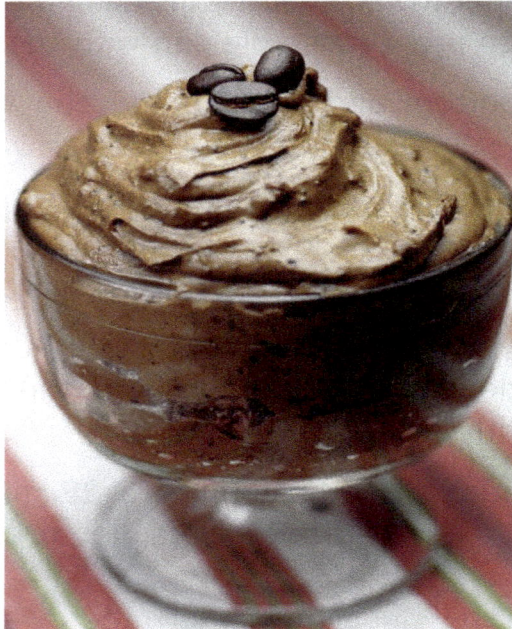

Coconut Brownies

Prep time: 15 min Cooking Time: 25 min serve: 2

Ingredients

½ cup coconut flour

2 tablespoons honey

½ cup butter

¼ cup raw cacao powder

1 egg

1/8 teaspoon acceptable sea salt

¼ teaspoon baking soda

¼ teaspoon pure vanilla extract

¼ cup dark chocolate chips

Directions

Line a 7-inch round pan with parchment paper. In a large bowl, combine the coconut flour, butter, honey, cacao powder, egg, salt, baking soda, and vanilla extract and stir well to create a thick batter.

Transfer the batter to the prepared pan and use your hands to press it evenly into the pan. Sprinkle with the chocolate chips and gently press them into the batter.

Pour 1 cup water into the Instant Pot and arrange the handled trivet on the bottom. Place the pan on top of the trivet and cover it with an upside-down plate or another piece of parchment to protect the brownies from condensation.

Secure the lid and move the steam release valve to Sealing. Select Manual/Pressure Cook to cook on high pressure for 15 minutes. When the cooking cycle is complete, let the pressure naturally release for 10 minutes, then move the steam release valve to venting to release any remaining pressure. When the floating valve drops, remove the lid.

Let the brownies cool completely in the pan before cutting and serving.

Nutrition Facts

Calories 302, Total Fat 26.4g, Saturated Fat 16.4g, Cholesterol 102mg , Sodium 321mg, Total Carbohydrate 14.8g, Dietary Fiber 0.7g, Total Sugars 12.9g, Protein 2.4g

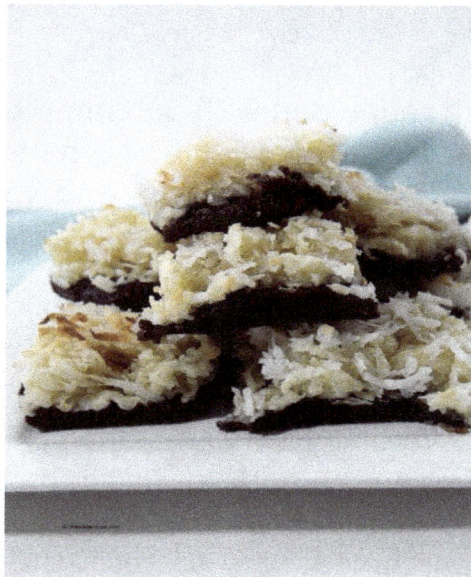

www.ingramcontent.com/pod-product-compliance
Lightning Source LLC
Chambersburg PA
CBHW062118040426
42336CB00041B/1849